WORKBOOK

to Accompany

Introduction to
SPORTS MEDICINE
&
ATHLETIC TRAINING

Robert C. France

Written by Gary R. Cannell

THOMSON

DELMAR LEARNING   Australia Canada Mexico Singapore Spain United Kingdom United States

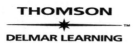

THOMSON

DELMAR LEARNING

Workbook to Accompany Introduction to Sports Medicine & Athletic Training
by Robert C. France
Written by Gary R. Cannell

Vice President, Health Care Business Unit:
William Brottmiller

Editorial Director:
Cathy L. Esperti

Acquisitions Editor:
Marah Bellegarde

Developmental Editor:
Darcy M. Scelsi

Editorial Assistant:
Erin Adams

Marketing Director:
Jennifer McAvey

Production Editor:
Bridget Lulay

Art and Design Coordinator:
Connie Lundberg-Watkins

Library of Congress Cataloging-in-Publication Number

ISBN 1-4018-1200-7

Notice to the Reader

CONTENTS

UNIT THREE

INJURY ASSESSMENT AND MANAGEMENT

PREFACE

This workbook has been developed from the textbook *Introduction to Sports Medicine and Athletic Training* with the goal of assisting students in maximizing the benefits derived from the textbook. The uniqueness of the textbook approach to sports medicine by the thorough incorporation of anatomy and physiology is completely integrated into the workbook as well. The organization of the workbook exactly mirrors that of the textbook, so the information and exercises of Chapter 12 of the workbook, for instance, originate from information presented in Chapter 12 of the textbook.

The workbook provides a review of textbook key concepts to help students grasp the main themes of each chapter, followed by a relatively detailed summary of textbook content presented in an organized outline form. The workbook then presents the student with vocabulary review exercises in the form of matching questions, crossword puzzles, and other word puzzles in an effort to emphasize the specialized vocabulary associated with the field of sports medicine. Anatomy identification exercises are provided in the appropriate chapters that emphasize terminology used throughout the field of medicine and show the anatomical relationships of one body part to another. Supplemental activities beyond those suggested by the textbook are also available in the workbook, including those that make use of the Internet, to further familiarize students with material presented in the textbook.

HOW TO BEST USE THE WORKBOOK

The key concepts listed at the beginning of each chapter of the workbook are primarily there as a convenience for students. In this one location, students will find a listing of all key concepts presented in the corresponding textbook chapter, without having to flip through several pages. This can be a particularly useful format for students studying for tests.

The best way to use the chapter outline provided in the workbook is while reading the textbook. Important information presented in the textbook can be highlighted on the outline as the student reads through each textbook chapter. Additionally, students can make notes to the side of the outline as the chapter is read or as information is presented in class, making the outline an even more useful workbook tool, while at the same time customizing textbook material to the teaching method and emphasis stressed by their own instructor.

The vocabulary review sections can be used most effectively as practice tests. By matching given definitions with word lists or by fitting words into crossword puzzle squares, the student can test his or her own ability to recognize the specialized terminology presented in the textbook. Since answer keys are provided only in the instructor's manual, these vocabulary review exercises can also be used as student assignments.

The anatomical identification exercises have two main purposes. One is simply to learn the names of the structures and their relationship to one another. The second purpose is to familiarize students with the overall shape of the structure. Coloring activities that accompany many of the diagrams in the workbook also force students to find the boundaries of specific structures within the human body. It is difficult to treat injuries of a muscle like the trapezius, for example, unless the caregiver knows where the trapezius begins and ends. While there are many ways to color a diagram, the best method seems to come from the use of colored pencils. Colored pencils have the advantage of light to dark shading depending on the pressure applied, the ability to be sharpened for the fine details within a diagram, and colored pencils do not bleed through the page.

The other activities suggested in each chapter are relatively specific to the subjects covered in that chapter. Often they will be used as assignment or classroom activities, but they can also provide ideas for independent study and research. For the Internet use, no specific web sites have been provided in the workbook. Instead, students are encouraged to use any of the various search engines available for the Internet. Web sites often come and go, but the ability to enter certain key words into a search engine can make the difference between getting useful, rather than useless, lists of information sources.

Used in conjunction with the material presented in *Introduction to Sports Medicine and Athletic Training*, the workbook will allow students to maximize their learning experience in this introduction to the exciting field of sports medicine.

CHAPTER 1

Sports Medicine:
The Multidisciplinary Approach
to Athletic Health Care

KEY CONCEPTS

- Sports medicine is a multidisciplinary approach to health care for those seriously involved in exercise and sport. Health care professionals from many disciplines are involved in the care of the athlete.

- The primary role of the health care providers involved in the athlete's care is to promote lifelong fitness and wellness, and encourage prevention of illness and injury. The professionals involved come from a variety of specialty areas such as physician assisting, physical therapy, nutrition, chiropractic, and sports psychology.

- Physician assistants work interdependently with a physician to aid in patient care duties.

- Parents play an active role in prevention and treatment of the athlete's injuries. Parents should maintain open communication with the athletic training staff regarding injury risk, athletic development, proper nutrition, and treatment of injuries.

OUTLINE

I. Sports medicine is a multidisciplinary approach for those seriously involved in sport, involving a variety of professionals, such as family and team doctors, physician assistants, certified athletic trainers, and physical therapists.

   A. Sports medicine was first recognized as a specialty in the twentieth century

   B. The American College of Sports Medicine was founded in 1954, promoting broadly trained physicians as an athlete's first contact when treating an injury.

   C. True sports medicine specialists have training that allows them to specifically address the needs of the athlete.

   D. Athletes today commonly participate in strenuous exercise and intense athletic competition, which inherently carries a high level of risk.

   E. With the expansion of professional athletics and the large number of participants at the college and high school levels, the importance of competition and performance has never been greater. Injury is often devastating to these individuals.

II. Professions associated with sports medicine and others associated with athletics make up the Athlete's Circle of Care.

A. Family and team doctor

1. Physicians promote lifelong fitness and wellness.

2. Two years of additional training through accredited subspecialty programs in sports medicine is common.

3. Additional training comes from continuing education and participation in sports medicine associations.

4. Ideally, a balance of care between the family doctor and the sports medicine physician specialist will provide the athlete with the most complete information and treatment.

B. Physician assistant

1. A recognized profession since the 1960s, the physician assistant provides the extension of consumer access to health services by extending the time and skills of the physician.

2. Duties include diagnostic and therapeutic patient care, and in most states, the ability to write prescriptions.

3. Many team doctors use the services of a physician assistant for patient care.

C. Physical therapist

1. Physical therapists specialize in a wide variety of areas in addition to sports medicine, including pediatrics, orthopedics, aquatic therapy, wound care, women's health, and many others.

2. Physical therapists can be found in a variety of health care facilities, such as hospitals, schools, and fitness facilities.

D. Physical therapy assistant

1. Patient care is provided along with the physical therapist.

2. Duties include developing treatment plans, documenting treatment progress, and modifying treatment established by the physical therapist as patients recover.

E. Chiropractor

1. Spinal manipulation is used instead of drugs or surgery to promote the body's natural healing process.

2. Chiropractors provide conservative management of neuromuscular disorders for back pain, neck pain, and headaches.

F. Massage therapist

1. One of the oldest methods of providing relief of pain and discomfort, massage today has become important in promoting wellness and reducing stress.

2. Massage therapists work along with physicians, nurses, and physical therapists in the promotion of health and healing.

G. Certified Strength and Conditioning Specialist/Personal Trainer

1. Fitness instructors monitor and modify the athlete's conditioning and strength training.

2. Certified Strength and Conditioning Specialist (CSCS) programs identify individuals who possess the knowledge and skills to design and implement safe and effective strength and conditioning programs.

H. A National Strength and Conditioning Association Certified Personal Trainer (NSCA-CPT) works one-on-one with clients in schools, health and fitness clubs, and even in a client's house.

I. Sports nutritionist

1. Nutritionists develop correct diets for athletic competitors and instruct athletes on supplements and dietary aids.

2. Improvement in performance can be achieved through special diets geared toward specific athletic events.

J. Sports psychologist

1. Sports psychologists are specially trained in athletic motivation and performance, using goal setting, imagery, and other techniques to give athletes an edge.

2. Sports psychologists can be found in clinical settings, educational institutions, private practice, and employed by professional sports teams.

K. Sports coach

1. At all levels, from young league competitions to professional sports teams, the coach teaches athletes how to compete without injury.

2. Good communication between the coach, athlete, and certified athletic trainer will ensure the best care for all athletes.

L. Parents

1. Parents should be actively engaged in the prevention and treatment of their child's injuries.

2. Parents can be directly involved with all sports medicine specialists, provide education to their children, and be active in providing proper nutrition and conditioning.

VOCABULARY REVIEW

Match the terms on the right with the statements on the left. Answers may be used once, more than once, or not at all.

_____ 1. Designs special diets to enhance athletic performance

_____ 2. The primary physician caring for the athlete

_____ 3. All individuals involved in the care of the athlete

_____ 4. A practitioner working interdependently with the physician

_____ 5. Provides pain relief through muscle manipulation

_____ 6. A specialist who designs and implements a safe and effective strength and conditioning program.

_____ 7. The study and application of scientific and medical knowledge to aspects of exercise and injury prevention.

_____ 8. Helps athletes recover through emotional support and motivation

_____ 9. Involved with the evaluation and rehabilitation of injury

_____ 10. Includes parents, certified athletic trainers, coaches, and many others.

A. Athlete's Circle of Care

B. Certified Strength and Conditioning Specialist (CSCS)

C. chiropractor

D. family and team doctor

E. massage therapist

F. National Strength and Conditioning Association Certified Personal Trainer (NSCA-CPT)

G. physical therapist (PT)

H. physical therapy assistant (PTA)

I. physician assistant (PA)

J. sports psychologist

K. sports medicine

L. sports nutritionist

ACTIVITIES

1. Research the educational requirements necessary beyond high school for each of the specialists on the sports medicine health care team.

_____

_____

_____

_____

_____

2. Select a sports medicine profession you would like to pursue after high school. Find a person in your community who is currently active in that profession, and find out what training he or she completed after high school and what training he or she is involved with as a professional to keep up with changes in the profession.

_____

_____

_____

_____

_____

ONLINE RESEARCH

■ Research your own state's laws regarding the certification and training of the various health care professions associated with sports medicine.

_____

_____

_____

_____

_____

■ Research the sports medicine programs available in schools similar to yours in your area. Compare and contrast these programs to the program at your school.

_____

_____

_____

_____

_____

CHAPTER 2

Athletic Training

■ Athletic training has a long history that dates back as far as the care Galen provided gladiators in ancient Rome. The recognition of athletic training as an allied health profession, however, did not come until 1991. As more and more people become involved in athletics, the field of athletic training is still evolving and developing. The future of athletic training promises growth.

■ The certified athletic trainer is a highly educated and skilled professional specializing in the prevention, treatment, and rehabilitation of injuries. The certified athletic trainer (ATC) works in cooperation with physicians and other allied health personnel.

■ Skills required for athletic training include problem solving, analyzing injuries, taping and bandaging, motor skills, communication, monitor rehabilitative programs, good judgment and decision-making, proficient knowledge in anatomy, physiology, biology, and advanced first aid, working with people. Certified athletic trainers must also be capable of demonstrating physical and rehabilitative movements, utilization of modalities and other training equipment, deductive reasoning skills, working well under stressful conditions, maintaining poise in emergencies, implementation of exercise and rehabilitation programs for athletes, and recording, organizing, and storing information on injuries and rehabilitation.

■ Certified athletic trainers have a wide variety of work settings available to them. These settings can range from working with athletes at various levels of competition from high school to college as well as in amateur to professional programs. ATCs can also work in clinic and industrial settings.

■ There are many professional organizations that support the field of sports medicine and athletic training. The most widely known is NATA, which is the organization that certifies most athletic trainers in the United States. Many states have their own professional organizations that promote the professional development of athletic trainers.

■ The Athlete's Bill of Rights sets standards and expectations for the fair treatment of any individual involved in sport or athletic competition.

■ Anyone who works outside the scope of practice and expertise can be found negligent and, therefore, liable for his or her actions. Certified athletic trainers should take appropriate precautions to prevent exposure to lawsuits.

OUTLINE

I. Athletic training is the rendering of specialized care to those individuals involved in exercise and athletics.

   A. Responsibilities include prevention, recognition, evaluation, care, and rehabilitation of injuries.

   B. The AMA recognizes athletic training as an allied health profession.

   C. Title IX prohibits discrimination on the basis of sex from participation in athletics in schools, greatly increasing the number of female athletes.

   D. ATCs are an integral part of the athletic health care team in secondary schools, colleges and universities, clinics, professional sports programs, and industrial settings.

   E. Certified athletic trainers typically work beyond the typical work day and often exceed 40 hours per week.

II. Certified Athletic Training

   A. ATCs must abide by the rules and procedures of their certifying organization and the state licensure or certification.

   B. Failure to act in accordance with these rules can result in disciplinary action or termination.

   C. The National Athletic Trainers' Association (NATA) is the largest certifying organization in the United States.

   D. Minimum education includes a bachelor's degree.

      1. Major areas of study are typically athletic training, physical education, or exercise science.

      2. Training includes human anatomy and physiology, biomechanics, exercise physiology, athletic training, nutrition, and psychology/counseling.

   E. A certification test is administered by the National Athletic Trainers' Association Board of Certification (NATABOC) consisting of multiple-choice questions, a practical evaluation of athletic training skills, and a written simulation test.

   F. Topics covered include the following domains of athletic training: prevention; recognition, evaluation, and assessment; immediate care; treatment, rehabilitation, and reconditioning; organization and administration; professional development and responsibility.

   G. Regional State and Local Trainers' Associations, found in most U.S. states, provide educational opportunities for certified athletic trainers, physicians, school administrators, athletic directors, coaches, parents, and athletes.

III. The Athlete's Bill of Rights is a series of standards that include the right to:

   A. have fun through sports.

   B. participate at a level commensurate with their maturity level.

   C. qualified adult leadership.

   D. participate in a safe and healthy environment.

   E. competent care and treatment of injuries.

   F. share the leadership and decision making of their sport.

   G. participate in a sport regardless of ability and income level.

   H. proper preparation for participation.

I. equal opportunity to strive for success.

J. be treated with dignity.

K. say "no."

IV. Liability and Risk Management

   A. Hippocratic Oath: "I will use treatment to help the sick according to my ability and judgment, but I will never use it to injure or wrong them."

   B. Anyone who works outside his or her scope of practice and expertise can be found negligent and, therefore, liable for his or her actions.

   C. To avoid possible lawsuits, certified athletic trainers should take certain precautions.

      1. Work within the scope of knowledge and expertise.
      2. Keep proper documentation and maintain accurate records.
      3. Follow proper training room rules and procedures.
      4. Always have adequate training room supervision.
      5. Keep in close contact with coaches, administration, and parents of athletes.
      6. Inspect practice and game facilities daily.
      7. Establish a return-to-play protocol.
      8. Involve the team physician in all aspects of the program.
      9. Establish an advisory program with members of all involved parties.
      10. Establish and practice an emergency action plan.

   D. Liability insurance can help avoid financial disaster.

VOCABULARY REVIEW

Matching

Match the terms on the right with the statements on the left. Answers may be used once, more than once, or not at all.

_____ 1. Prohibits discrimination on the basis of sex from participation in athletics in schools receiving federal funds

_____ 2. Policies and standard for fair treatment of athletes

_____ 3. A professional involved in the prevention, recognition, evaluation, and care of injuries

_____ 4. Any area of health care that contributes to or assists the professions of physical medicine, dentistry, optometry, pharmacy, and podiatry

_____ 5. An ancient declaration that has become a fundamental part of the practice of medicine

A. allied health profession
B. Athlete's Bill of Rights
C. athletic training
D. certified athletic trainer (ATC)
E. ahtletic training student aide
F. Hippocratic Oath
G. Title IX

Word Search

The following word search puzzle includes 14 specialized words or terms used in Chapter 2. See if you can find them all.

```
R   N   S   D   L   P   D   J   E   T   Z   N   W   C   T
E   A   K   E   N   A   N   E   I   K   O   I   O   G   N
H   T   D   Q   T   M   W   T   I   I   W   D   M   P   E
A   A   P   C   D   A   L   S   T   L   E   O   A   F   M
B   B   Z   A   F   E   R   N   U   O   L   K   N   I   S
I   O   W   B   I   Z   E   C   F   I   X   A   N   C   S
L   C   W   X   I   V   I   C   O   U   T   V   P   Z   E
I   N   X   W   E   A   O   E   U   P   A   K   M   M   S
T   A   F   R   V   N   I   B   R   C   P   Z   E   L   S
A   W   P   C   D   L   I   A   B   I   L   I   T   Y   A
T   W   T   U   C   B   Z   W   J   V   E   C   H   P   A
I   A   C   T   Z   D   A   U   C   M   M   K   P   Z   T
O   T   S   T   H   G   I   R   F   O   L   L   I   B   A
N   G   K   V   Y   R   T   I   B   L   Z   Z   C   R   N
U   N   E   U   O   C   R   E   N   I   A   R   T   Y   Z
```

ALLIED	ASSESSMENT	ATC
BILLOFRIGHTS	CODEOFCONDUCT	HIPPOCRATES
LAWSUIT	LIABILITY	NATA
NATABOC	PREVENTION	REHABILITATION
TITLEIX	TRAINER	

ACTIVITY

1. Research the use of the Hippocratic Oath among the modern health professions.

_____

_____

_____

_____

_____

ONLINE RESEARCH

■ Research how your favorite sports teams use certified athletic trainers: how many are employed and what their responsibilities are. Compare the use of certified athletic trainers among the different sports. For instance, how does basketball differ from baseball?

_____

_____

_____

_____

_____

CHAPTER 3

The Central Training Room

KEY CONCEPTS

- The modern central training room should be adequately designed to promote the proper care of both male and female athletes. The room should meet the following specifications: appropriate size for needs; adequate lighting, plumbing, electricity, as well as ventilation and heating; telephone access, office space, a wet area, a taping area, a treatment area, and an exercise and rehabilitation area.

- All athletic training staff must preserve the confidentiality of privileged information and should not release such information to a third party not involved in the patient's care.

- Most sports medicine budgets are tight and often require creative measures to make ends meet. Supplies must be ordered to adequately stock the training room that can be used in a reasonable time frame. Consideration must be given to product expiration dates, identifying patterns of purchasing, and establishing relationships with vendors for special pricing.

- There are three general modalities used in the central training room: mechanical, involving manipulation of the muscles in the body; thermal, involving the use of heat or cold; and electrical, involving the use of electrical stimulation and other electrical devices.

- Equipment and supplies must be well stocked in the medical kits as well as on site for games and practices. Common supplies necessary to have on hand are bandages, splinting devices, crutches, ice packs, water, and first aid equipment.

- Federal OSHA regulations are put in place for the protection and safety of workers who are at risk to exposure of bloodborne pathogens. OSHA mandates an exposure control plan be on hand, the training of staff on bloodborne pathogens, documentation and reporting of all exposures, that personal protective equipment be available to staff, availability of the hepatitis B vaccine to all at-risk staff, special containers to be used for biohazardous materials and sharps, that the staff follows Standard Precautions, and proper disinfection techniques be used to clean tools and work surfaces.

OUTLINE

I. Design of the Central Training Room
   A. The central training room must be easily accessible to both male and female athletes.
   B. Size of the room
      1. A typical large high school (1,500–2,000 students) will have about 25% of the population involved in athletics.
      2. An ideal room for a large high school would be 1,200 square feet, though most tend to be in the range of 400–800 square feet.
   C. Adequate lighting will allow for proper examinations and treatments.
   D. Plumbing
      1. Water needs include a sink, ice machine, whirlpool, and hydrocollator.
      2. Drainage is necessary for the floor in wet areas.
      3. Planning should include a dishwasher and washing machine.
   E. An adequate number of electrical outlets for special equipment and modalities, including ground fault interrupters (GFI) for all areas near water.
   F. Ventilation is necessary to prevent problems with humidity, and heating levels should be appropriate for typical athletic attire.
   G. Telephone access is important for safety and emergencies.
      1. Both a building line and a long distance line are recommended.
      2. Emergency numbers must be clearly posted.
      3. Cell phone and pager numbers of all training staff should be available with instructions on whom to contact in an emergency.
   H. Storage, including locked cabinets, should be sufficient to accommodate unanticipated needs.
   I. An office within the training room is necessary to secure personal information, including information stored on a computer, private consultations, and examinations.
   J. The wet area should consist of the refrigerator, ice machine, whirlpool, and hydrocollator.
   K. The taping area will be the most utilized space in the training room.
      1. There should be at least six tables, separated by 18" to 24" of space between them.
      2. Tables can be padded and covered with vinyl or covered with countertop laminate.
   L. At least two treatment tables, similar to the taping tables, are also recommended.
   M. With adequate space, an exercise area should include an exercise bike, and an elliptical trainer for rehabilitation of various areas of the body.
II. Operating the Central Training Room
   A. The program director is responsible for the overall operation of the Sports Medicine program and facility.
      1. Responsibilities include staffing the central training room and managing equipment, inventory, budgets, recordkeeping, athletes, coaches, parents, and school administration.
      2. The program director should distribute the workload to other staff members.

III. Rules and Procedures

    A. Injury management policy

        1. All injuries must be reported to the certified athletic trainer as soon as possible for documentation and follow-up.

        2. The athletic training staff will preserve the confidentiality of all information associated with the athlete's condition.

        3. The certified athletic trainer will be responsible for the final decision on an athlete's playing status.

        4. Athletic training student aides will keep the coach informed of the athlete's status.

    B. Housekeeping

        1. Surfaces in contact with people must be cleaned at least daily with a disinfectant, after each use for high use areas.

        2. Whirlpools are cleaned before and after each use.

        3. Sinks, countertops, towels, hydrocollator covers, and instruments must be cleaned daily.

        4. Handwashing is necessary before and after each treatment.

    C. Dress code and personal hygiene

        1. Men wear a collared shirt, women a professional shirt, tucked into pants.

        2. Pants or shorts, khaki, should be worn.

        3. Socks with functional shoes (no open toe or sandals) should be required.

    D. Budgeting

        1. Create a list of consumable supplies and a separate list of reusable supplies.

        2. Track all supplies; monitor staff involved in the ordering process and inventory.

        3. Develop a working relationship with a vendor who understands the needs of the facility.

        4. Reviewing past purchases and training room treatment logs will allow the development of a purchasing pattern.

        5. Ask for free samples to test products before mass purchases.

        6. Because of limited shelf lives, some supplies will have to be ordered several times each year.

    E. Appropriately supplied medical kits, from fanny packs to large kits requiring wheels for transport, will ensure prompt and adequate treatment of athletes.

        1. Equipment should be inspected daily to ensure proper working order.

        2. Game site equipment

            a. Vacuum splints allow for air extraction, conforming the splint to the injury without exerting unnecessary pressure or impairing circulation.

            b. Air splints add air to increase pressure surrounding an injury site.

            c. SAM® splints are lightweight and can immobilize almost any bone in the body, including the neck.

            d. Other splints include padded wooden splints, articulated splints, and small splinting materials used for fingers.

        3. Crutches, including the new HOPE crutch that allows the user to comfortably walk using less energy than traditional crutches, allow for patient mobility when weight cannot be placed on leg structures or hips.

F. General first aid supplies

    1. Consumable supplies are many and varied.

    2. Nonconsumable supplies include blankets, braces, CPR devices, penlights, scissors, sharks, tweezers, nail clippers, slings, and splints.

    3. Other training room supplies include a refrigerator, ice machine, tables, benches, carts, desks, computers, exercise equipment, rehabilitation items, stretchers, immobilizers, and neck collars.

G. Therapeutic modalities, whose purpose is to help the athlete promote healing and mobility, include electrical stimulation, heat (hydrocollator), ice, Transcutaneous Electrical Nerve Stimulation, ultrasound, and whirlpool. Some require permission and supervision of a physician.

H. Water is necessary in the form of water bottles, water tables, cups, or pressurized containers to keep athletes properly hydrated. Containers must be sterilized daily.

IV. OSHA (Occupational Safety and Health Administration) Standards

A. Federal regulations have been developed for employees whose jobs may put them at risk to bloodborne pathogens.

B. Definitions

    1. Bloodborne pathogens—pathogenic microorganisms that are present in human blood and can cause disease in humans

    2. Contaminated—the presence of or reasonable anticipated presence of blood or other potentially infectious materials on an item or surface

    3. Contaminated sharps—any contaminated object that can penetrate the skin

    4. Standard precautions—an approach to infectious control

C. Standard precautions

    1. Wear vinyl or latex gloves whenever touching biohazardous material such as open skin, blood, body fluids, or mucus membranes. Do not reuse gloves.

    2. Wash hands with soap and water immediately after being exposed to blood or body fluids, even if gloves were worn.

    3. Wash all surfaces soiled with blood or body fluids, using a 10% household bleach solution or a commercially available disinfectant.

    4. Place all sharps in a special puncture-resistant sharps container.

    5. Place all discarded medical waste in a container labeled "Biohazardous Waste."

    6. When outdoors, medical waste is disposed of into a red biohazard bag, which is later discarded into the training room's biohazardous waste container.

    7. Do not allow athletes to share contaminated towels.

    8. Towels and clothing that have been contaminated must be placed into a biohazard bag and placed in the laundry basket.

    9. Be sure all athletes' wounds are well covered before practice and competition.

    10. If any training staff has an open wound, especially on the hand, avoid providing first aid care for injuries involving blood or body fluids, unless absolutely necessary, being sure to wear vinyl or latex gloves.

D. Disinfecting procedures

    1. All equipment and environmental and working surfaces shall be cleaned and decontaminated after contact with blood or other potentially infectious materials.

2. Disinfection should be done with a chemical germicide registered with the Environmental Protection Agency or a 10% bleach-to-water solution.

3. Cleaning spills
    a. Use standard precautions.
    b. Dispose of sharps in a sharps container.
    c. Use an absorbing pad, such as a paper towel, or an absorbing powder, such as cornstarch, depending on spill size.
    d. Place spilled material in a biohazardous waste container.
    e. Decontaminate using a disinfectant over the entire spill area.
    f. Remove soiled protective equipment and place in a labeled biohazardous waste container.

4. Daily cleaning procedures
    a. Clean all surfaces.
    b. Wipe all surfaces with a clean, dry towel.
    c. Wet the inside of the whirlpool with water, wet a towel with whirlpool disinfectant, rinse the inside of the whirlpool with cold water, dry with a clean towel.
    d. Place instruments, using clean hands, in an instrument tray filled with an approved instrument cleaning solution for 10 minutes, rinse with warm water, dry, and replace.
    e. Wash hands.

VOCABULARY REVIEW

Crossword Puzzle

Identify the terms described in the puzzle clues, then write the letters in the boxes. (Many terms are more than one word.)

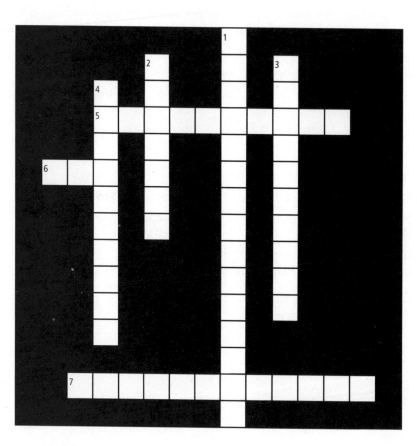

Across

   5. a therapeutic treatment such as ultrasound and TENS _____

   6. a mini circuit breaker that responds to shorts or contact with water _____

   7. a multipurpose facility that accommodates athletic training needs _____

Down

   1. instruments that can penetrate the skin _____

   2. a therapeutic treatment that may involve a hydrocollator or ice packs

   _____

   3. a therapeutic treatment that involves muscle manipulation _____

   4. a portable storage container; for example, fanny packs _____

Word Search Puzzle

Several medical kit supplies can be found among the letters of the word search puzzle. How many can you find? (Many terms are more than one word.)

```
R  A  O  O  Q  S  E  U  C  D  B  E  R  V  T
O  S  D  G  F  O  N  S  X  A  L  E  F  I  R
S  C  B  H  R  O  G  N  N  A  T  G  K  Z  O
S  I  B  H  E  O  O  D  S  E  S  S  G  X  L
E  S  M  Y  X  S  A  T  M  B  N  U  W  V  L
R  S  M  C  F  I  I  O  P  E  B  C  P  A  E
P  O  F  B  D  C  M  V  L  O  O  U  F  C  R
E  R  M  S  W  R  B  T  E  K  W  S  J  I  G
D  S  Z  R  E  B  C  K  L  T  L  D  K  F  A
E  Q  A  H  S  A  W  E  Y  E  A  F  E  M  U
U  P  T  H  T  W  H  X  G  Q  N  P  A  R  Z
G  P  O  N  V  X  T  W  U  P  E  N  E  N  E
N  Q  O  S  E  V  O  L  G  X  E  T  A  L  T
O  C  B  I  O  H  A  Z  A  R  D  B  A  G  S
T  A  N  A  L  G  E  S  I  C  S  A  R  U  R
```

ADHESIVETAPE   ANALGESICS   BANDAIDS
BIOHAZARDBAGS   CONTACTLENSKIT   ELASTICWRAP
EYEWASH   FOOTPOWDER   LATEXGLOVES
ROLLERGAUZE   SCISSORS   THERMOMETER
TONGUEDEPRESSOR

ACTIVITIES

1. Attend and participate in training sessions that show the proper technique for cleaning the various types of equipment in the training room. Demonstrate what you have learned by showing your trainer how to clean equipment properly.

_____

_____

_____

_____

_____

2. Start going to athletic practices and games with experienced student trainers to observe what they do on the job, particularly looking for what the trainers do to prevent the spread of bloodborne pathogens. Write a report on what you observe, relating your observations to the topics covered in Chapter 3.

_____

_____

_____

_____

_____

ONLINE RESEARCH

- Use various web searches to explore local and state regulations regarding athletic and student trainers, what they can do, and what they are not allowed to do. Search for local guidelines on the prevention of spreading disease through disinfection and other cleaning techniques.

_____

_____

_____

_____

_____

- Research local guidelines regarding the athletic training room. Identify size and spacing requirements that must be taken into consideration during the design of athletic training rooms.

_____

_____

_____

_____

_____

CHAPTER 4

The Athletic Training Student Aide Program

KEY CONCEPTS

■ Athletic Training Student Aides (ATSAs) not only gain valuable experience in a clinical setting, but also enable the sports medicine director to spend more time addressing the needs of the entire program. An ATSA program benefits the student by allowing him or her to gain knowledge and skills toward a career in the health care industry. The certified athletic trainer benefits from an ATSA program that allows more administrative time.

■ Many states have included sports medicine as a vocational class, which has made it eligible for state education dollars. Funding can also come from base education funds, school district allocations, associated student body dollars, and athletic booster clubs or grants.

■ Expectations of student athletic training aides and the athletic training director are high. ATSAs should be motivated, in good academic standing, able to make and carry through on commitments, and be positive role models. Some of the daily responsibilities of the ATSAs are to maintain equipment and supplies; maintain the training room facility; communicate with athletes, the certified athletic trainer, and coaches; and assist in the care and treatment of injuries under the supervision of the certified athletic trainer.

■ Evaluations are most useful when changes can be made periodically as the year progresses. Evaluations should be made in the areas of individual ATSAs, overall sports season, end-of-year evaluation, and evaluation of the program director.

OUTLINE

I. Athletic Training Student Aide (ATSA)

  A. ATSAs are very important to both high school and college athletic training programs

    1. ATSAs gain valuable clinical experience.

    2. Sports medicine directors can spend more time addressing the needs of the entire program.

    3. Students desiring a career in medicine are able to gain valuable knowledge while still in high school.

    4. Well-trained student aides can assist in most aspects of the athletic training program.

II. Organizing a First-Class Program

    A. Certified athletic trainers must be able to develop, maintain, and promote an environment that provides appropriate prevention, assessment, treatment, and rehabilitation of athletic injuries.

    B. Outcomes must be clearly defined to both coaches and administrators of the school.

    C. Keep communication lines open to coaches, athletic training staff, athletes, and parents, to alleviate concerns over the role of the athletic training program.

    D. Program staff

        1. The program director determines how many ATSAs are required in the program, as well as their training and educational requirements.

        2. The size of the school, number of sports covered by the athletic training program, and overall objectives help determine numbers of ATSAs.

    E. Program funding

        1. Vocational funding provides one of the major sources for many of today's ATSA programs.

        2. Basic education dollars can be made available by allowing the sports medicine class to give students either physical education or science credit.

        3. Other sources include school district allocations, associated student body dollars, and athletic booster clubs.

III. A Model Program

    A. Success depends on the training and involvement of students in the program.

    B. A three-year program, with sports medicine taught the final two periods of the day, has been particularly successful.

        1. The first period is designated as the lab science, where the student learns advanced first aid and CPR, anatomy and physiology, kinesiology, biomechanics, and sports psychology.

        2. During the second period, students are in the athletic training room working with athletes, for the practical session of the class.

    C. Students must always be supervised by a certified athletic trainer.

    D. Many states have guidelines that regulate student aide responsibility.

    E. A three-year program offers the possibility of increasing student responsibility throughout their time in high school.

        1. First-year students can work as apprentices, learning from second- and third-year students.

        2. Second-year students take on more leadership responsibilities.

        3. Third-year students assume the role of "head ATSAs," in charge of all their sports' organizational needs, setting schedules, and checking paperwork before the program director gives approval.

    F. Students should take an active role as soon as possible in the program. Successful programs that retain students for the full three years are those that allow students to have ownership in their program.

IV. Student Expectations

    A. When everyone has a say in how the program will operate, expectations will be easily achieved.

B. Students need to be highly motivated, willing to make a long-term commitment, academically successful, on time, able to work well with others, self-starters, willing to do more than asked, and positive role models.

C. Responsibilities of ATSAs

1. Stock the first aid kit, check equipment, stock the ice chest, fill water bottles.

2. Check the injury list from the previous practice or game.

3. Communicate with the certified athletic trainer and coaches.

4. Help with the treatment of injuries and taping (under direct supervision).

5. Clean training room before and after practices and games.

6. Update the supply list; check out equipment.

7. Maintain a proper training room atmosphere; review the season with staff and the program director.

D. Daily duties

1. ATSAs must wear proper clothing or a uniform.

2. ATSAs must be active during practices and games, watching what is happening at all times.

3. Following the athletic training schedule is no different than a schedule for a job. Students must commit to the program.

E. Head ATSA responsibilities

1. Responsible for all aspects of his or her sport.

2. Set the training schedule one week in advance.

3. Conduct weekly meetings with first- and second-year students, communicating expectations.

4. Communicate with coaching staff daily; program directors, parents, and administration as needed.

5. Check for completed paperwork, and complete the final report at the end of the season.

F. Incentives such as ATSA of the Month, hourly accomplishments, school letters, and recognition at end-of-season banquets can help motivate students to do their best.

V. Evaluation

A. Evaluation should be an ongoing process, but is especially useful when changes are made during the year.

B. Successful programs continually evolve through self and outside evaluation. Constructive evaluation encourages learning and allows the program to run more efficiently.

C. Areas of evaluation should include individual ATSAs, head ATSAs, the overall sports season, coach evaluations of ATSAs and the athletic program, an end-of-year evaluation, and an evaluation of the program director.

VOCABULARY REVIEW

Word Search

The following word search puzzle includes terms that relate to the responsibilities of ATSAs and head ATSAs. See how many you can find.

```
H  F  E  C  T  A  M  G  T  J  M  Q  I  T  K
A  V  S  M  N  R  T  E  F  X  F  S  S  I  R
V  K  K  N  M  W  O  M  E  A  Z  K  D  K  O
E  C  B  J  A  K  E  P  O  T  P  Y  C  D  W
F  E  A  M  I  A  K  R  E  S  I  K  R  I  R
U  H  A  P  H  Q  E  K  Z  R  P  N  Z  A  E
N  C  I  B  S  V  R  U  J  Z  L  H  G  T  P
E  T  A  C  I  N  U  M  M  O  C  A  E  S  A
W  A  T  E  R  B  O  T  T  L  E  R  N  R  P
Q  E  W  U  G  G  N  I  P  A  T  K  L  I  E
X  H  T  U  W  O  O  P  W  Q  C  R  M  F  F
T  R  E  A  T  M  E  N  T  O  W  C  B  F  D
U  O  K  Z  D  P  V  A  T  A  V  A  S  H  E
R  Z  C  J  U  P  V  S  E  N  H  O  L  Q  R
T  S  I  L  Y  R  U  J  N  I  X  O  D  S  G
```

ATMOSPHERE	CHECK	COMMUNICATE
FINALREPORT	FIRSTAIDKIT	HAVEFUN
INJURYLIST	MEETINGS	PAPERWORK
REVIEW	STOCK	TAPING
TREATMENT	UPDATE	WATERBOTTLE

ACTIVITIES

1. At your school, observe how ATSAs accomplish their responsibilities. What are the differences in responsibility as the ATSA becomes more experienced and more highly trained?

_____

_____

_____

_____

_____

2. Get involved with your school's ATSAs, assisting them with their duties as much as your current level of training allows. Write a summary of your experiences, particularly noting the ATSA responsibilities, how they accomplish them, and how much time is spent with the various tasks required of them.

_____

_____

_____

_____

_____

ONLINE RESEARCH

■ Research local and state guidelines regarding Athletic Training Student Aides (ATSAs). Compare responsibilities outlined in Chapter 4 with the duties allowed in your school.

_____

_____

_____

_____

_____

CHAPTER 5

Emergency Preparedness:
Injury Game Plan

KEY CONCEPTS

- Each athletic organization has a duty to develop an emergency plan that can be implemented immediately, and to provide appropriate health care to all participants.

- A written emergency action plan (EAP) is important so that a systematic approach can be followed in an emergency. This will help to avoid mistakes and inadequate treatment.

- An EAP should be tailored to the program for which it is written. It should outline the emergency needs in the following four areas: emergency personnel, emergency communication, emergency equipment, and transportation.

- The athletic training staff should have clearly defined roles in an emergency. These roles should encompass immediate care for the athlete, retrieval of emergency equipment, activation of the EMS system, and directing the EMS scene.

- When activating EMS, the following information must be readily available: the name, address, and phone number of the caller; the number of athletes injured; the condition of the injured; care and treatment being provided at the scene by the athletic training staff; specific directions to the scene; and any other information asked for by the dispatcher.

- The difference between a defined medical emergency and a nonemergency is the potential threat of loss of limb or life. An injury, no matter how minor, should be reported to the certified athletic trainer.

- Emergency medical cards are valuable to the athletic training staff because they allow the staff to have all important contact information at their fingertips. Emergency medical cards also permit the athletic training staff to treat, and provide access to emergency care for, an injured minor athlete in the event the parents or guardians are unavailable.

OUTLINE

I. Emergency Preparedness

    A. Certified athletic trainers must be properly equipped and trained for any medical crisis or disaster that may arise.

    B. Necessary for emergency preparedness is an emergency action plan, proper coverage, emergency equipment and supply maintenance, appropriate medical personnel, and continuing education.

II. The Emergency Action Plan

    A. Written action plans deal with injuries in a systematic, logical manner that helps avoid missteps and mistakes.

    B. Emergency Action Plan (EAP)

        1. The EAP should be customized to fit the needs of the organization, and should be practiced and reviewed at least once every year to familiarize everyone involved with the process.

        2. The EAP should specify needs for emergency personnel, communication, equipment, and transportation.

        3. Roles of emergency personnel should be clearly outlined.

        4. All members of the athletic training staff are responsible for knowing and being able to implement the emergency plan.

        5. Immediate care for the injured athlete should be provided by the most qualified member of the athletic staff present.

        6. One member of the staff should be assigned to activate the Emergency Medical Service (EMS) system, the response system called upon in the event of a medical crisis or traumatic injury.

    C. Activating the EMS system

        1. Good working relationships between the athletic training staff and emergency medical personnel help establish rapport and define roles in an emergency.

        2. A working telephone must be available, along with a backup plan for communication.

        3. Clearly communicate to EMS the name, address, and phone number of the caller; the number of athletes injured; the condition of the injured; care and treatment currently being provided; specific directions to the scene; and any other information requested by the dispatcher.

    D. Emergency equipment

        1. All equipment necessary to handle emergency situations must be readily available and in good working condition.

        2. Individuals providing care to the athlete must be knowledgeable in the use and application of the equipment.

    E. Transportation

        1. EMS providers and an ambulance should be on standby at any event where there is a high risk of traumatic injury.

        2. The onsite ambulance should have clear access to the site so that entering and exiting can be done without delay.

        3. Athletes with unstable injuries should never be transported in a vehicle that is not appropriately equipped.

III. Identifying a Medical Emergency
   A. Defined medical emergencies consist of breathing cessation, severe bleeding, no pulse, concussion with loss of consciousness, neck or spinal injury, fractures, dislocations, eye injuries, severe asthma attack, heat-related illness, or any injury causing signs of shock.
   B. Nonemergencies include injuries that do not threaten life or limb, such as abrasions, minor cuts, strains, sprains, minor concussions without the loss of consciousness, or contusions.
   C. All injuries, no matter how minor, should be reported to the athletic training staff.
IV. Emergency Medical Cards
   A. Each athlete must have an up-to-date emergency information profile on record.
   B. Emergency medical cards should include parent/guardian contact information, medical information that may be of use in an emergency, hospital preference, doctors' phone numbers, parental permission for treatment and transportation.

VOCABULARY REVIEW

Matching

The following vocabulary terms are associated in some way with the statements or conditions listed. Identify which term goes with which statement or condition. (Terms may be used more than once.)

_____ 1. An outline of emergency steps taken

_____ 2. Possible life-threatening injury

_____ 3. The ambulance or equipped emergency vehicle

_____ 4. Abrasions

_____ 5. Heat-related illness

_____ 6. Concussion without loss of consciousness

_____ 7. Specifies the roles of emergency personnel

_____ 8. Being properly trained

_____ 9. Activation often involves communication with a dispatcher

_____ 10. Severe bleeding

_____ 11. Sprains

_____ 12. Being properly equipped

_____ 13. Personalized to the needs of the organization

_____ 14. Includes information of transportation

_____ 15. Includes personnel trained in life support

A. defined medical emergency

B. emergency action plan (EAP)

C. emergency preparedness

D. EMS system

E. nonemergency

ACTIVITIES

1. Examine one of your school's emergency cards. What information is provided? What does the emergency card let certified athletic trainers at your school do that could cause problems if there were no emergency cards? What else would you include on the card that might be helpful in case of emergency?

_____

_____

_____

_____

_____

2. If possible, participate in a simulated emergency performed by local EMS services. Report on what your experience was and how the EMS personnel and others responded to your situation.

_____

_____

_____

_____

_____

ONLINE RESEARCH

■ Research emergency action plans from other high schools, colleges, and universities in your area. Explain how they differ from your school's EAP and why those differences exist (funding, availability of services, personnel, etc.).

_____

_____

_____

_____

CHAPTER 6

The Pre-Participation
Physical Examination

KEY CONCEPTS

■ The pre-participation physical examination (PPE) is needed to help identify athletes at risk for specific types of injuries and identify preventative techniques to avoid injury. The PPE opens the door to a working relationship between the athlete and the physician. The overall goal of the PPE is to maintain the health and safety of the athlete.

■ In an office-based examination, the athlete's family physician completes a thorough evaluation of the athlete's physical status. In a station-based examination, the athlete is evaluated by many physicians or specialists, each responsible for one aspect of the complete physical evaluation.

■ The components of the pre-participation physical examination include baseline medical history; height, weight, blood pressure; assessment of eyes, ears, nose, and throat; and evaluation of the heart, abdomen, genitalia, skin, and musculo-skeletal system.

■ The physician must consider any potential problems that may put the athlete at risk for injury and weigh those against the potential risks involved in the sport in which the athlete wants to participate. Based on this analysis the physician must determine if the athlete is able to compete fully, able to compete only after training and rehabilitation, or unable to compete due to the risk being too high.

■ All information contained on the PPE is confidential and must be treated with the strictest of confidence.

OUTLINE

I. The Pre-Participation Physical Examination (PPE)

    A. Over the years, the PPE has gone from a cursory examination to a comprehensive overall assessment of an athlete's health and ability to perform a sport at the highest level.

    B. The primary goal of the PPE is to help maintain the health and safety of the athlete. Other goals include:

        1. Determination of the athlete's general health

        2. Disclosure of defects that may limit participation

        3. Detection of conditions that may predispose the athlete to injury

4. Determination of the optimal level of performance

5. Classification of the athlete according to individual requirements

6. Fulfillment of legal and insurance requirements

7. Evaluation of the level of maturation of younger athletes

8. Evaluation of fitness and performance for possible improvement prior to participation

9. Provision of opportunities to compete for students with specific health issues that may preclude a blanket approval.

10. Provisions of opportunity to counsel youths regarding personal health issues

11. Entry of the athlete into the local sports medicine environment, thereby establishing a doctor-patient relationship

C. The PPE should take place at least six weeks before the beginning of the sports season so if musculoskeletal problems are found, there will be time to rehabilitate and strengthen the areas of concern.

D. The station-based pre-participation examination

1. Many athletes can be examined in the same setting, often for lower cost.

2. The athlete is examined by sports medicine specialists.

3. Stations include medical history and basic measurements of blood pressure, height, weight, eyesight.

4. Specialists often include family physicians, orthopedic specialists, physical therapists, certified athletic trainers, podiatrists, and pediatricians.

5. Difficulties with the station-based PPE include finding volunteer medical specialists and a location for the examination.

E. The office-based pre-participation physical examination

1. The family physician, the usual evaluator, has access to the complete medical history of the athlete.

2. The setting is quiet and allows for the discussion of multiple health issues.

3. Immunization history is available and can easily be updated.

II. Components of the Pre-Participation Physical Examination

A. A complete medical history will identify approximately 75% of all problems affecting athletes. The recommended baseline history includes medical conditions and disease, surgeries, hospitalizations, medications, allergies, immunization status, menstrual history, pulmonary status, neurological status, musculoskeletal status, and injuries or illness since the last exam.

B. The recommended components of the PPE include height, weight, pulse, blood pressure, eyes, ears/nose/throat, heart, abdomen, genitalia (males only), skin, and musculoskeletal.

III. Clearance

A. Clearance, the term used for physician permission for athletic participation, is divided into three categories.

1. Unrestricted clearance

2. Clearance after completion of further evaluation or rehabilitation

3. No clearance for certain types of sports or for all sports

B. When an abnormality is found, the physician must consider several questions.

   1. Does the problem place the athlete at risk for injury?

   2. Is another participant placed at risk of injury because of the problem?

   3. Can the athlete safely participate with treatment?

   4. Can limited participation be allowed while treatment is being completed?

   5. If clearance is denied only for certain sports or sports categories, in what activities can the athlete safely participate?

C. Sports are classified based on degree or level of contact and strenuousness, which may result in clearance for some, but not all sports.

III. Recordkeeping

A. Physical forms are completed and signed by the physician.

B. Information from the PPE is available to coaches, trainers, and the athletic director.

C. All information contained on the PPE is confidential and must be treated with the strictest of confidence by storing the forms in the certified athletic trainer's or athletic director's office under lock and key.

D. All PPE forms should be kept and stored for a minimum of seven years after the athlete graduates or leaves the school.

VOCABULARY REVIEW

Matching

Match the terms on the right with the statements on the left. Terms may be used more than once.

_____ 1. It is usually difficult to find an adequate facility

_____ 2. Allows for the use of specialists

_____ 3. Has the advantage of low cost

_____ 4. Usually completed by the athlete's family physician

_____ 5. Individual athlete medical histories are readily available

_____ 6. Originally consisted of a short (often less than five minutes physical)

_____ 7. The overall goal is to help maintain the health and safety of the athlete.

_____ 8. Many athletes can be taken care of at once.

_____ 9. A quiet setting allows for more doctor-patient discussion.

_____ 10. Immunization deficiencies can be easily updated.

_____ 11. Should take place at least six weeks before the sports season.

A. office-based PPE

B. pre-participation physical examination (PPE)

C. station-based PPE

Word Search

Several contact and limited-contact sports can be found among the letters of the word search puzzle. How many can you find? (Many terms are more than one word.)

```
H  O  R  S  E  B  A  C  K  R  I  D  I  N  G
T  I  C  E  S  K  A  T  I  N  G  C  F  S  L
F  A  T  G  U  R  G  Z  F  G  R  H  M  K  L
I  V  C  Z  N  N  U  E  L  O  C  A  G  A  A
E  C  C  K  I  I  N  G  S  G  R  N  N  T  B
L  P  E  X  L  C  D  S  B  T  V  D  I  E  D
D  I  O  H  I  E  C  R  I  Y  J  B  F  B  N
H  B  A  N  O  O  F  A  A  M  W  A  R  O  A
O  J  G  L  U  C  L  O  I  O  I  L  U  A  H
C  O  R  N  N  A  K  I  O  Y  B  L  S  R  M
K  M  T  F  R  O  D  E  O  T  V  W  U  D  A
E  R  B  T  R  M  J  G  Y  Q  B  C  O  I  E
Y  C  S  L  L  A  B  T  E  K  S  A  B  N  T
L  L  A  B  T  O  O  F  G  A  L  F  L  G  S
C  H  E  E  R  L  E  A  D  I  N  G  O  L  H
```

BASKETBALL	BOXING	CHEERLEADING
CROSSCOUNTRY	FENCING	FIELDEVENTS
FIELDHOCKEY	FLAGFOOTBALL	HANDBALL
HORSEBACKRIDING	ICEHOCKEY	ICESKATING
MARTIALARTS	RODEO	RUGBY
SKATEBOARDING	SNOWBOARDING	SURFING
TACKLEFOOTBALL	TEAMHANDBALL	WINDSURFING

ACTIVITIES

1. Research the importance of blood pressure, especially regarding athletic performance. Describe how blood pressure is measured and what is happening to the arteries of the arm when a nonelectronic sphygmomanometer is used.

_____

_____

_____

_____

_____

2. Obtain a nonelectronic sphygmomanometer and stethoscope from your teacher to practice taking your own blood pressure and the blood pressure of others in your class until you are comfortable in your knowledge of what you hear through the stethoscope and what it means.

_____

_____

_____

_____

3. Measure your own blood pressure every day for a week and calculate an average. How does this compare to the average for your age and sex?

Average Blood Pressure				
	SYSTOLIC		**DIASTOLIC**	
Age (Years)	**Men**	**Women**	**Men**	**Women**
10	103	103	69	70
12	106	106	71	72
14	110	110	73	74
16	118	116	73	72
18	120	116	74	72
20–24	123	116	76	72
25–29	125	117	78	74
30–34	126	120	79	75
35–39	127	124	80	78
40–44	129	127	81	80
45–49	130	131	82	82
50–54	135	137	83	84
55–59	138	139	84	84
60–64	142	144	85	85
65–69	143	154	83	85
70–74	145	159	82	85

_____

_____

_____

_____

_____

4. Fill out the Sports Qualifying Physical Examination form used at your school. Write your own evaluation of how clearly the questions are asked. Are there any confusing portions of the form? If so, suggest a way that the information can be gathered more clearly. How much of the information did you know compared to how much you had to ask of others (parents, physician, etc.)?

_____

_____

_____

_____

_____

ONLINE RESEARCH

■ Choose a fall sport, a winter sport, and a spring sport; then research, through the Internet, the most common injuries athletes in your chosen sports suffer and how debilitating these injuries are. If the injuries do keep the athlete from participating for long periods of time, identify what they must do to regain full function once they do return to the sport.

_____

_____

_____

_____

_____

CHAPTER 7

Prehabilitation and Preseason Conditioning

KEY CONCEPTS

- Prehabilitation decreases the chance of injury by addressing areas of concern or deficit identified before participation in a sporting event. A program can be implemented to strengthen and develop these areas, thus reducing the chance of injury during participation.

- Preseason conditioning allows athletes to gradually build up to a level of activity that will be expected of them on the playing field. By starting slowly, the body is allowed to adjust to the new demands. Once the body has accommodated, the athlete can once again increase the demand on the body. By working incrementally to get the body adjusted, the athlete can prepare for the demands of the season.

- In isometric exercise, the muscles maintain a constant length throughout the contraction. This is a good type of exercise to target an exact area of weakness due to an injury. In isotonic or dynamic exercise, there is movement of the joint during muscle contraction. This type of exercise helps improve blood circulation, strength, and endurance. Isokinetic exercises use machines to control the speed of the contraction within a range of motion. These exercises provide muscle overload at a constant, preset speed and full range of motion.

- Manual resistance training is done with a partner. The partner adds resistance to a lift, allowing the muscles to fatigue, and then releases enough resistance so the lifter can finish the range of motion. Circuit training uses 6 to 10 strength exercises completed one after another, performed for a specific number of repetitions or time period. Individualized training programs allow an athlete to work with a personal trainer to develop a program that allows him or her to meet specific goals. A variety of exercise types can be used.

- Progressive resistance training allows the body to adapt to the increased demand placed upon it through training. The rate and type of strength gain is determined by four factors:
    1. Overload is the overwork of muscles at tensions close to their maximum
    2. Specificity is the targeting of a particular muscle group alone
    3. Reversibility is the characteristic of muscles that causes decreases in strength and mass with disuse
    4. Individual differences also account for an individual's ability to strengthen certain muscles at a particular rate. Genetics have a strong influence on strength gain.

- Stretching and flexibility decrease the chances of injury. Stretching allows the athlete to actually lengthen the muscles, resulting in an increased range of motion. Therefore, joints and limbs can move further before an injury occurs.

- Cardiorespiratory training conditions the heart and other muscles to use oxygen more efficiently. This allows the athlete to perform for longer periods of time.

OUTLINE

I. Prehabilitation

    A. A preventative management program with the goal of preventing injury

    B. This program addresses concerns or deficits recognized by the athlete's family physician or other sports medicine specialist prior to sports participation.

II. Preseason Conditioning

    A. Whenever athletes start a fitness program, or after they take an extended period of time off, their bodies need time to adjust to the new stresses and demands.

    B. Preseason conditioning focuses on developing the athlete in the off-season.

        1. The conditioning program should begin six to eight weeks prior to sports participation to allow the body to gradually adapt to the demands to be placed on it.

        2. Sports medicine physicians, certified athletic trainers, and qualified youth coaches should prescribe a preseason conditioning program and provide athletes with information on the type, frequency, intensity, and duration of training.

III. Strength training

    A. Strength training is a highly adaptive process whereby the body changes in response to increased training loads.

        1. Adaptation requires a systematic application of exercise stress sufficient to stimulate muscle fatigue without injury.

        2. If muscle is worked beyond its normal limits, it adapts by becoming larger (hypertrophy).

        3. If a muscle is worked less than normal, it becomes smaller (atrophy).

        4. The purpose of progressive resistance exercise is to allow the body to adapt to the increased demand placed upon it.

    B. Overload

        1. Muscles increase in size and strength when they are forced to contract at tensions close to maximum.

        2. Muscles must be overloaded at a progressively increased rate.

        3. The ideal number of repetitions is between four and eight, done in multiple sets of three or four.

        4. Proper rest intervals between sets allow muscles to recover from exertion and prepare for the next work interval.

    C. Specificity

        1. Muscles adapt specifically to the nature of the work performed, an attribute known as specificity.

        2. When muscles contract, they recruit different types of motor units to carry out the contraction.

            a. Slow-twitch fibers are recruited for low-intensity activities such as jogging, and are relatively fatigue-resistant.

            b. Fast-twitch fibers are used for high-speed or high-intensity activities, such as weightlifting, and fatigue more rapidly.

        3. Increases in strength, including rehabilitation after injury or surgery, are very specific to the type of exercise, which should be as close as possible to the desired movements of the activity.

4. Muscle fiber type appears to play an important role in determining success in some sports, such as distance running and sprints, but not in others, such as shot-putting.

D. Reversibility

1. Muscles atrophy with disuse, immobilization, and starvation.

2. Slow-twitch fibers will typically atrophy faster than fast-twitch fibers, an important factor to consider when designing a rehabilitation program after immobilization.

E. Individual differences

1. Some differences in the strength gain rate are due to the relative predominance of fast- and slow-twitch motor units in muscles.

2. Fiber composition is genetically determined, although a good training program can make up for genetic deficiencies.

F. Stretching and flexibility

1. Stretching, moving joints beyond their normal range, is useful for injury prevention as well as injury treatment.

2. Range of movement is increased due to increasing the length of the muscles, which means that limbs and joints must move further before an injury occurs.

3. Warming up is an essential component of stretching by increasing heart rate, blood pressure, and respiratory rate, consequently increasing oxygen and nutrient delivery to the muscles.

4. Flexibility is the ability of a joint to move freely through its full range of motion.

   a. An active person tends to be more flexible than an inactive person.

   b. Females tend to be more flexible than males

   c. Older people tend to be less flexible than younger people

   d. Flexibility is as important as muscular strength and endurance

   e. To achieve flexibility in a joint, the surrounding muscles must be stretched.

5. Types of Stretching

   a. Static stretching is a gradual stretching of a muscle through the muscle's entire range of motion, done slowly until a pulling sensation occurs.

   b. Ballistic stretching involves a rhythmic, bouncing action, largely discounted today due to its tendency to increase the incidence of injury.

   c. Proprioceptive neuromuscular facilitation (PNF) involves a combination of contraction and relaxation of the muscles, requiring an initial isometric contraction against maximum resistance at the end of the range of motion, and is designed to be done with a qualified assistant.

G. Isometric exercise

1. Muscles contract, but there is no movement in the affected joints.

2. Muscle fibers maintain a constant length throughout the entire contraction.

3. Isometrics are often used for rehabilitation because the exact area of muscle weakness can be isolated, and strengthening can be administered at the proper joint angle.

4. Blood pressure also increases rapidly, so individuals with circulatory problems and high blood pressure should avoid strenuous isometric exercises.

H. Dynamic or isotonic exercise

1. Movement of the joint does occur during the muscle contraction.

2. Manual resistance is accomplished using a training partner, sometimes called a spotter.

   a. The spotter adds enough resistance to allow the lifter to fatigue the muscles, and then release enough resistance so that the lift can be completed.

   b. Advantages include minimal equipment is required, the spotter can help control technique, workouts can be completed in less than 30 minutes, and training can be done anywhere.

   c. A disadvantage is getting an inadequately trained spotter. Both the lifter and spotter should be trained so that the exercise is safe and effective.

I. Isokinetic exercise

   1. Machines are used to control the speed of contraction within the range of motion.

   2. Machines such as the Cybex and Biodex provide isokinetic results; they are generally used by physical therapists and are not readily available to the general population.

J. Circuit training

   1. Six to ten strength exercises are completed, one after another until all are done.

   2. Each exercise is performed for a specific number of repetitions or a specific period of time before moving on to the next exercise, with a brief rest time in between.

   3. If more than one circuit is to be completed, the circuits will be separated by a longer rest period.

IV. Special Individualized Programs

   A. Personal trainers can assist in strength training, cardiovascular fitness, speed and endurance work, and body composition. Personal trainers should be certified or have proven knowledge and expertise.

   B. Certified athletic trainers are allied health professionals who have a considerable knowledge of anatomy and physiology. They can be found at many high schools and most colleges and universities.

V. Cardiorespiratory Conditioning

   A. Also known as aerobic or endurance training, cardiorespiratory conditioning refers to activities that put an increased demand on the lungs, heart, and other body systems.

   B. Large muscle groups are used for activities such as walking, jogging, swimming, cross-country skiing, or cycling.

   C. The goal of cardiorespiratory conditioning is to train the heart and other muscles to use oxygen more efficiently, allowing the athlete to perform exercise for longer periods of time.

   D. Results include an increase in heart size, thus lowering the resting heart rate and blood pressure. Also oxygen transfer rates are more efficient and resting metabolism increases.

   E. Other benefits include reduced fatigue, improved self-confidence, improved muscle strength and tone, increased endurance, reduced stress levels, reduced body fat, and improved overall physical and mental health.

VOCABULARY REVIEW

Crossword Puzzle

Identify the terms described in the puzzle clues, then write the letters in the boxes. (Many terms are more than one word.)

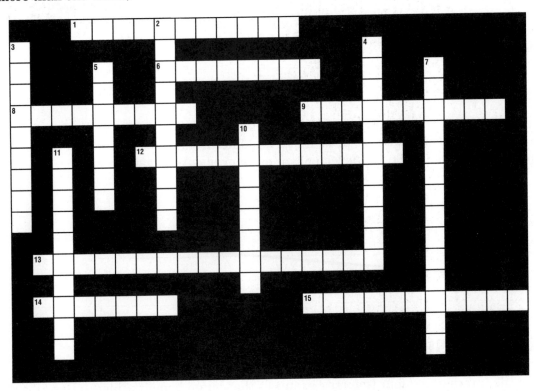

Across

1. the ability of a joint to move freely through its full range of motion

   _____

6. a condition where muscles are progressively overworked at an increased

   _____

8. a motor nerve plus all the muscle fibers it stimulates _____

9. the moving of joints beyond the normal range of motion _____

12. the process of muscle atrophy due to disuse, immobilization, or starvation

   _____

13. a type of training that puts an increased demand on the lungs, heart, and other body systems _____

14. a type of training that uses 6 to 10 strength exercises completed one after another for a specific time _____

15. the ability of particular muscle groups to respond to targeted training

   _____

Down

2. a type of exercise in which a machine is used to control the speed of contraction

   _____

3. tension in the muscle increases but it does not move _____

4. an increase in muscle size

   _____

5. a decrease in muscle size resulting in weakness and wasting away

   _____

7. the process of restoring function through programmed exercise _____

10. an activity that causes the muscle to contract and shorten _____

11. the systematic application of exercise stress

   _____

ACTIVITIES

1. Research the anatomy and physiology of the motor unit. Draw the basic structure of a motor unit.

_____

_____

_____

_____

_____

2. Describe how motor units in the larger muscles of the body, like the biceps brachii in the upper arm or the quadriceps of the upper leg, differ from motor units in the smaller muscles that control finger movements or eye movements. Create an anatomical drawing that shows these differences.

_____

_____

_____

_____

_____

ONLINE RESEARCH

■ On the Internet find four isometric exercises that might benefit athletes. Describe the exercises fully and the benefits they might have for athletes in a specific sport.

_____

_____

_____

_____

■ Research the terms _hypertrophy_ and _atrophy_. Describe changes actually taking place within the muscle to cause an increase or a decrease in its size. Identify the long-term consequences of muscle atrophy in terms of its ability to contract.

_____

_____

_____

_____

CHAPTER 8

Nutrition and the Athlete

OUTLINE

I. Nutrition

    A. Nutrition is defined as the process by which a living organism assimilates food and uses it for growth and for replacement of tissues.

    B. Proper nutrition can reduce the likelihood of injury and allow the athlete to perform at a higher level.

II. Energy

    A. Energy is the power used to do work or to produce heat or light.

    B. Energy can be changed from one form to another, but cannot be created or destroyed.

    C. Living plants are able to convert solar energy into the chemical energy of carbohydrates, fats, and proteins by a process called photosynthesis.

    D. Animals get their energy from the chemical energy contained in plants and other animals.

        1. Energy maintains body functions, such as breathing, heartbeat, and heat production.

        2. Energy is necessary for active movement; for example, muscle contraction.

        3. Energy is used for growth and repair.

    E. Energy is measured in calories, the energy needed to raise the temperature of one gram of water from 14.5 to 15.5 degrees Celsius (C).

        1. One kilocalorie (kcal) equals 1,000 calories.

        2. One food calorie is equal to one kilocalorie.

        3. Carbohydrates and proteins contain four food calories per gram, while fats provide nine food calories per gram.

III. Food Components

    A. The human body must have a balanced diet consisting of carbohydrates, proteins, fats, vitamins, minerals, water, and fiber.

    B. Carbohydrates

        1. Carbohydrates in the form of glucose are the body's primary source of fuel.

        2. Sugars are considered to be simple carbohydrates and starches complex carbohydrates, although both end up as glucose after digestion.

        3. Complex carbohydrates in the form of fruits, vegetables, and whole grains are often accompanied by vitamins and minerals, as well as fiber.

        4. Excess glucose is stored in the liver and muscles as glycogen or converted to fat for storage in fat cells.

        5. Glucose levels in the blood are controlled by hormones insulin and glucagon, produced in the pancreas.

            a. Insulin stimulates the body cells and liver to take glucose from the blood, and glucagon causes glucose to be released into the blood as the liver converts glycogen back into glucose.

            b. The balance of insulin and glucagon keeps the blood sugar levels relatively constant. Diabetes is a condition of having little or no insulin produced by the pancreas.

6. About 45% to 50% of daily calories come from carbohydrates, mostly from complex carbohydrate sources.

   a. The daily diet should include 6 servings of grains, 3 servings of vegetables, and 2 servings of fruits.

   b. The average American adult gets about twice as many calories from simple carbohydrates (sugars) than recommended.

7. The most basic sugar is the monosaccharide, which includes glucose, fructose, and galactose.

   a. Disaccharides are composed of two monosaccharides, such as sucrose (table sugar), which is composed of one glucose and one fructose chemically bonded together.

   b. Polysaccharides, such as starch, glycogen, and cellulose, are composed of hundreds to thousands of glucose molecules chemically bonded together.

C. Protein

1. Proteins form one of the body's main structural elements and are found in every cell.

2. Proteins are important components of muscles, connective tissue, skin, organs, blood, some hormones, antibodies, and enzymes.

3. Each protein is composed of varying combinations of 20 different building blocks called amino acids, many of which are provided to the body by the breakdown of dietary protein during digestion.

   a. Nine of these amino acids are considered "essential" because they must be provided by the diet, while the 11 others are considered "nonessential" because they can be manufactured by the body.

   b. A "complete protein" is a food that contains all of the essential amino acids, whereas an "incomplete protein" is a food that is low in one or more of the essential amino acids.

   c. While most plant proteins are incomplete, a well-balanced vegetarian diet can provide the body with all needed amino acids.

4. Cells reassemble amino acids obtained from the diet and from the liver into proteins the body can use.

5. The average adult's requirement for protein is considered to be 0.8 grams per kilogram of body weight.

D. Dietary fat

1. Fat is a carrier of fat-soluble vitamins, provides essential fatty acids, is an important source of stored energy, and provides insulation against the loss of body heat.

2. Fatty acids are important components of fats.

   a. Saturated fatty acids are usually solid at room temperature and have been associated with increased risk of cancer and heart disease when eaten in excess.

   b. Monounsaturated fatty acids are liquid at room temperature and have been less associated with disease unless hydrogenated, as in margarine, which makes them solid at room temperature.

c. Polyunsaturated fatty acids, the primary fat found in seafood, are liquid or soft at room temperature. Polyunsaturated fatty acids, such as linoleic acid and alpha-linolenic acid, are considered essential fatty acids because they are required in the diet and used in the body for cell structure and producing some hormones.

d. Trans fatty acids are made when unsaturated fatty acids are hydrogenated to make margarines, shortening, and other solid fats.

3. No more than 10% of an individual's daily calories should come from saturated fats, with no more than 30% from all fats.

E. Vitamins

1. Vitamins are complex organic substances that the body needs in small amounts for a variety of different body functions.

2. Insufficient amounts of vitamins in the body will result in deficiency disorders that have specific symptoms.

3. Fat-soluble vitamins are stored in the body's fat reserves and released as the body needs them.

a. Taking large doses can be toxic.

b. Vitamins A (retinol), D (calciferol), E (tocopherol), K_1 (phytonadione), K_2 (menaquinones), and K_3 (menadione) are all fat-soluble vitamins.

4. Water-soluble vitamins are not stored in great amounts in the body and must be replenished regularly.

a. Excess water-soluble vitamins are excreted by the body in urine and do not reach toxic levels.

b. Water-soluble vitamins include vitamin B_1 (thiamine hydrochloride), B_2 (riboflavin), B_6 (pyridoxine hydrochloride), C (ascorbic acid), nicotinic acid (niacin) and nicotinamide (niacinamide), B_{12}, and folic acid.

F. Minerals

1. Minerals are essential parts of enzymes. They participate in regulating many physiological functions including transporting oxygen to cells, providing a mechanism for muscle contraction, and allowing nerve cells to conduct signals.

2. Most minerals are found in a variety of foods, although deficiencies can occur.

G. Water

1. Water is a most important nutrient, since a loss of just 2% to 3% of body weight will impair performance and a loss of 7% to 10% can be fatal.

2. The kidneys play an important role in regulating the body's water balance.

3. Water helps regulate body temperature, transport nutrients, eliminate toxins and waste products, and maintain proper metabolism.

4. To maintain proper hydration, six to eight glasses of fluids should be consumed each day; more when active.

a. Prehydrate by drinking a glass or two of fluids within an hour of exercise to help the body cope with immediate water loss due to perspiration, increased respiration, and so on.

b. During and after the activity, drink as much liquid as possible. Restricting water intake during a practice or game is not only dangerous, it will hamper performance.

5. Sports drinks
    a. Today's sports drinks contain sugar, minerals such as potassium and sodium, and water, and sometimes vitamins. Sports drinks with ephedra (ma huang) should be avoided due to dangerous side effects.
    b. Sports drinks are particularly useful during long, hard workouts lasting more than one hour; otherwise water is more than adequate.
    c. The real advantages of sports drinks come from their sugar content, allowing muscles to gain energy and delay fatigue.

H. Dietary fiber
    1. Dietary fiber is the indigestible component of plant material that humans consume.
    2. Fiber keeps the digestive tract running smoothly. Soluble fiber helps lower cholesterol levels, while insoluble fiber adds bulk to intestinal contents, preventing constipation and making it easier for the intestines to eliminate waste.
    3. It is suggested that the normal diet consist of approximately 25 grams of fiber per day.

IV. Daily Values
    A. The Daily Value is a U.S. Food and Drug Administration guide to help consumers use food label information in planning their overall diet.
    B. Daily Reference Values (DRVs) are based on the National Academy of Sciences' 1998 Recommended Dietary Allowances and Dietary Reference Intakes (DRIs).
    C. DRVs for energy-producing nutrients are based on the number of calories consumed per day, with 2,000 calories per day as the reference.
        1. The amount of fat is based on 30% of daily calories.
        2. Saturated fat is based on 10% of calories.
        3. Carbohydrates are based on 60% of calories.
        4. Protein is based on 10% of calories.
        5. Fiber intake is based on 11.5 grams per 1,000 calories of fat, carbohydrates, and proteins.
    D. DRVs for some nutrients represent the uppermost limit that is considered desirable, since excesses can cause health problems.
        1. Total fat should be less than 65 grams.
        2. Saturated fat should be less than 20 grams.
        3. Cholesterol should be less than 300 milligrams.
        4. Sodium should be less than 2,400 milligrams.

V. The Food Guide Pyramid
    A. The Food Guide Pyramid was designed by the U.S. Department of Agriculture (USDA) and the Department of Health and Human Services (HHS) as an easy way to show the groups of foods that make up a good diet, identifying proper proportions by the relative size of each group in the pyramid.
    B. The Food Guide Pyramid also indicates the number of recommended daily servings for each group.

C. USDA and HHS Guidelines
  1. Aim for a healthy weight.
  2. Be physically active each day.
  3. Let the Pyramid guide your food choices.
  4. Choose a variety of grains daily, especially whole grains.
  5. Choose a variety of fruits and vegetables daily.
  6. Keep food safe to eat.
  7. Choose a diet that is low in saturated fat and cholesterol and moderate in total fat.
  8. Choose beverages and foods to moderate your intake of sugars.
  9. Choose and prepare foods with less salt.
  10. If you drink alcoholic beverages, do so in moderation.

D. Other cultures base their food pyramids on foods commonly eaten by their people, just as the Food Guide Pyramid from the USDA is based on what Americans eat. All food pyramids, however, emphasize eating plenty of whole grain products, vegetables, and fruits, and recommend physical activity.

E. Food groups
  1. Breads, cereals, rice, and pasta make up the bottom of the pyramid, providing complex carbohydrates, vitamins, minerals, and fiber.
  2. Vegetables, the next level up, provide vitamins A, C, folate, minerals such as iron and magnesium, and are a good source of fiber.
  3. Fruits provide vitamins A, C, and minerals like potassium.
  4. Meat, poultry, and fish provide protein, B vitamins, iron, and zinc.
  5. Milk products provide protein, vitamins, and minerals such as calcium.
  6. Fats, oils, and sweets—the top and smallest part of the pyramid—while necessary in small amounts, should be limited, even though some nutrients found here are important.

VI. Nutritional Quackery

A. New dietary supplements are marketed each day, often developed and sold without any scientific research to support their claims of benefits, and without proving no harmful side effects. These are treated by the FDA as foods and are not evaluated for safety and effectiveness.

B. Individuals and companies promoting these dietary supplements prey on the innocent, unsuspecting athlete who is eager for an edge on the competition or who may be looking for an easy alternative to hard work and training.

C. Before taking any product, the athlete should check with someone who has nutritional training for advice. The best protection against nutritional quackery is to be an informed consumer.

VII. Making the Weight

A. One of the most important aspects of fitness and athletic performance is controlling weight.

B. Gaining weight, without gaining fat, is only possible through weight training programs. Without a weight training program and increased energy expenditure, excess caloric intake will be converted to fat.

C. Losing weight can be accomplished by restricting calorie intake or exercise or both.

1. Minimum caloric intake for females should not go below 1,000 to 1,200 calories per day, 1,200 to 1,400 calories for males.

2. The best way to lose weight is through a combination of a moderate diet and exercise.

3. Exercise can increase cardiorespiratory endurance and result in a gain in strength and increased flexibility, all positive changes to a person's overall health.

4. It is always important to check with the family physician before beginning any weight loss or gain program.

VIII. Disordered Eating

A. Disordered eating patterns include anorexia nervosa, bulimia nervosa, and binge eating, all dangerous behaviors that can result in serious health problems.

B. Out of all athletes with disordered eating behaviors, 10% are male, many of whom are wrestlers. Extreme weight loss measures aimed at losing a few pounds as quickly as possible to make their weight are not only unhealthy, but can be deadly.

C. The female athlete triad

1. The female athlete triad consists of disordered eating, amenorrhea, and osteoporosis, and is especially prevalent among gymnasts, figure skaters, divers, and dancers, swimmers, and runners.

2. Symptoms include eating alone, trips to the bathroom during and after meals, use of laxatives, fatigue, anemia, depression, and eroded tooth enamel due to frequent vomiting.

3. Treatment involves education, nutrition, determining contributing factors, and being under the care of a medical specialist trained in disordered eating.

D. Anorexia nervosa

1. Anorexia nervosa is a psychophysiological disorder, usually occurring in young women, that is characterized by an abnormal fear of becoming obese, a distorted self-image, a persistent unwillingness to eat, and severe weight loss.

2. Self-induced vomiting, excessive exercise, malnutrition, and amenorrhea often accompany the disorder.

3. Symptoms include at least a 15% loss of normal body weight, loss of appetite, loss of menstruation, fatigue and dizziness, constipation, and abdominal pains.

4. Complications connected with anorexia nervosa are starvation, dehydration, muscle and cartilage deterioration, osteoporosis, irregular or slow heartbeat, and heart failure.

E. Bulimia

1. Bulimia is an eating disorder, common among women of normal or nearly normal body weight, characterized by episodic binge eating followed by feelings of guilt, depression, and self-condemnation.

2. Bulimia is often accompanied with measures taken to prevent weight gain, such as self-induced vomiting, the use of laxatives, dieting, or fasting.

3. Symptoms include fluctuations in weight, dental cavities from vomiting stomach acid, dehydration, fatigue and dizziness, constipation and abdominal pains, swelling of salivary glands, and irregular or absent menstruation.

4. Complications associated with bulimia include stomach ulceration, bowel damage, inflammation or tearing of the esophagus, laxative addiction, tingling hands and feet, and electrolyte imbalances that can lead to heart failure.

IX. Special Diets

A. Before embarking on any special diet, the athlete should talk with the family doctor, nutritionist, certified athletic trainer, or health professional.

B. Pregame meal

1. Energy for the game actually comes from muscle glycogen stores that are built up by consuming high carbohydrate meals every day, not just the pregame meal.

2. The pregame meal helps supplement muscle glycogen stores and prevents a low blood sugar level, with its accompanying light headedness, fatigue, and low concentration.

3. The pregame meal should be eaten three to four hours before the game, with foods high in carbohydrates and fluids. Grain products, vegetables, and fruits are the best choices because they are digested quickly and are readily available for fuel.

4. Protein intake should be moderate, and foods that are high in fat, sugar, or contain caffeine should be avoided altogether.

X. Calculating "Ideal" Weight for Athletes

A. Body mass index (BMI) is a reliable indicator with some limits of total body fat. BMI = Weight (lb.) ÷ Height (in.) ÷ Height (in.) × 703

B. Normal weight should have a BMI range of 18.5 to 24.9, overweight 25 to 29.9, and obesity 30 or greater.

C. Another method is to use a weight chart that compares others of the same age and gender, based on a national average.

VOCABULARY REVIEW

Crossword Puzzle

Identify the terms described in the puzzle clues, then write the letters in the boxes. (Many terms are more than one word.)

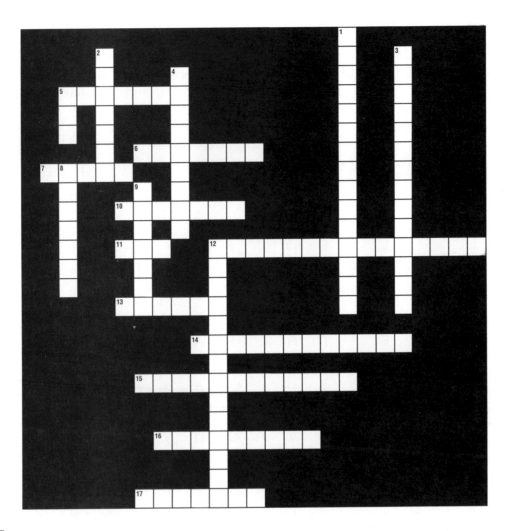

Across

5. an eating disorder characterized by binge eating _____
6. anorexia _____
7. the indigestible component of plants that is consumed by humans _____
10. an inorganic substance that participates in physiological processes _____
11. a nutrient that is a source of energy and insulates the body _____
12. fats with limited hydrogen as in those found in fish _____
13. the power used to do work or to produce heat or light _____
14. an essential nutrient that provides the primary source of fuel _____
15. a double sugar like sucrose, maltose, and lactose _____
16. the process by which living organisms assimilate food for growth _____
17. an essential nutrient containing nitrogen that helps the body grow _____

Down

1. fats missing some hydrogens such as vegetable, peanut, and olive oils _____
2. the unit of energy _____
3. the simplest form of a carbohydrate sugar _____
4. fats that contain the maximum number of hydrogens _____
5. the medical standard used to define obesity (abbr.) _____
8. a hormone that lowers the level of glucose in the blood _____
9. a complex organic substance that contains no energy _____
12. starch, cellulose, or glycogen _____

Word Search

Several foods that are high in soluble or insoluble fiber can be found among the letters of the word search puzzle. How many can you find? (Many terms are more than one word.)

```
J  P  E  P  G  Q  W  Q  V  Z  T  F  O  O  P
W  U  J  V  S  L  D  G  Q  V  Y  L  M  G  O
W  J  D  J  L  P  C  O  J  P  L  A  C  Y  T
B  S  U  Y  I  F  A  A  V  B  D  P  N  A  A
Q  C  A  D  T  K  A  T  N  A  U  Y  E  A  T
X  T  E  J  N  E  Q  B  S  P  S  H  N  A  O
O  J  G  S  E  I  R  R  E  B  W  A  R  T  S
F  C  Z  L  L  O  U  A  R  E  N  U  O  Y  K
Y  Y  P  Q  C  P  R  N  L  A  P  R  C  Y  I
L  P  C  C  S  M  T  O  B  X  R  J  P  E  N
A  S  O  A  H  E  H  V  P  A  U  Y  O  X  N
V  L  M  F  F  W  F  H  C  A  N  I  P  S  I
I  R  Z  X  Q  C  C  P  J  L  E  M  G  F  Y
L  O  F  G  O  B  E  F  H  G  S  W  Q  C  D
R  F  M  T  P  C  X  K  I  J  A  N  Q  U  H
```

APPLE	BANANA	BRAN
BROCCOLI	CARROT	LENTILS
OATBRAN	PEAR	PEAS
POPCORN	POTATOSKIN	PRUNES
SPINACH	STRAWBERRIES	WHOLEWHEAT

ACTIVITY

1. Select four canned or boxed meals that you and/or your family eat on a regular basis. Try to select meals that have some carbohydrates, fats, and protein. (Examples might be canned stew, chili, microwave dinners, and boxed lunches.) Take the nutrition label from these foods. Compare what you would eat from each of these meals with the nutritional guideline recommendations listed in the textbook. Pay attention to the serving size listed on the nutrition guide. If you normally eat the equivalent of two servings, you must double all other values on the chart to accurately represent what you are putting into your body.

_____

_____

_____

_____

_____

ONLINE RESEARCH

■ Find three examples of nutritional quackery on the Internet and explain how these products are promoted to appeal to athletes.

_____

_____

_____

_____

_____

■ Find a specific case study describing one of the eating disorders described in this chapter. Explain how the person described fits the average description of those most susceptible to the condition you are researching.

_____

_____

_____

_____

_____

CHAPTER 9

Dietary Supplements and Performance Enhancers

KEY CONCEPTS

■ Dietary supplements are products that are believed to enhance the diet. They come in a variety of forms. The effects of dietary supplements on the body will vary based on the supplement used and the amount used. Megadoses of dietary supplements can be harmful and lead to toxicity.

■ There is a vast array of dietary supplements on the market today. They consist of vitamins (for example, vitamin E, B-complex, and vitamin C); minerals (for example, zinc, iron, and sodium); herbs (for example, St. John's Wort, ginkgo biloba, and ginseng); and other naturally occurring substances (for example, glucosamine and chondroitin).

■ Performance enhancers are substances that athletes use because they believe the substances will enhance athletic performance, strength, and endurance. Athletes may experiment with performance enhancers because they are striving and being pushed to win no matter what the cost.

■ To maintain ethics in athletics and fairness in competition, many organizations have banned the use of performance enhancers and monitor the athletes in the organizations for use of these substances. The two largest organizations that monitor use of performance-enhancing drugs by athletics are the National Collegiate Athletic Association (NCAA) and the International Olympic Committee (IOC).

■ Athletes need to understand the inherent dangers and risks associated with the use of dietary supplements and performance enhancers. Some of these substances can be harmful to the athlete's overall health. Knowledge about these substances will help athletes make sound, informed decisions.

■ The athletic code of ethics places emphasis and value on honesty, integrity, good sportsmanship, and proper conduct.

OUTLINE

I. Popular Nutritional Supplements

    A. A dietary supplement is a product, other than tobacco, intended to enhance the diet that bears or contains one or more of the following ingredients: vitamins, minerals, amino acids, herbs, and other botanical substances.

    B. Vitamins

        1. Normally, a healthy person who eats a balanced diet will get all the vitamins needed.

        2. Vitamins are classified as natural or synthetic. The body uses both in the same way.

        3. Vitamins do not provide energy and they do not build muscles. They help release the energy from the carbohydrates and fats people ingest.

        4. The only disorders that can be cured by vitamins are those caused by vitamin deficiencies.

        5. If vitamin supplements are thought to be necessary by the athlete, a physician or registered dietitian should be consulted first.

    C. Minerals

        1. Minerals are inorganic elements or molecules that do not provide energy, but in their role as body regulators, can contribute to the production of energy from carbohydrates and fats.

        2. Concentrated forms of minerals should be used only on the advice of a physician.

    D. Herbal supplements

        1. Medicinal herbs have provided some of the oldest medicines, however the effectiveness of many herbs has not been proven. Since the FDA treats herbal products as dietary supplements, manufacturers of these products are not required to demonstrate the safety or effectiveness of their products before they are put on the market, as drug manufacturers do.

        2. The composition of herbal products can vary greatly from one batch to another.

    E. Glucosamine

        1. Glucosamine is naturally produced by the human body to maintain cartilage in the joints.

        2. Glucosamine has been proven as an effective treatment for osteoarthritis and as an aid in the recovery of some sports injuries.

        3. Side effects include stomach problems, heartburn, and diarrhea. People with heart problems or high blood pressure should consult a physician first. Glucosamine should not be taken by people using heart medications or insulin.

    F. Chondroitin

        1. Chondroitin is a naturally occurring substance found in human and animal cartilage.

        2. It has proven abilities to treat osteoarthritis.

        3. Anticoagulant users should consult their physicians before using chondroitin.

II. Performance Enhancers

    A. An ergogenic aid is any agent that enhances energy utilization, including energy production and efficiency.

B. Anabolic steroids

1. Anabolic steroids are manmade substances chemically related to male sex hormones.

2. Anabolic steroids are available legally only by prescription.

3. Athletes and others who abuse anabolic steroids often take them for a specific period of time, then quit for a while, then start again (cycling), and they will combine several types (stacking) in hopes of minimizing negative effects.

4. Major side effects of anabolic steroid abuse include liver tumors and cancer, jaundice, fluid retention, high blood pressure, increased bad cholesterol (LDL), and decreased good cholesterol (HDL).

5. Other side effects include kidney tumors, severe acne, and trembling. Also, in males, testicle shrinkage, reduced sperm count, infertility, baldness, breast development, and increased risk of prostate cancer may occur. Females may suffer from growth of facial hair, male-pattern baldness, menstrual cycle cessation, clitoral enlargement, and a deepening voice. The adolescent's skeleton may mature prematurely, permanently stopping growth in height.

6. Various mental conditions are associated with anabolic steroids, such as aggression, mood swings, depression if the steroids are stopped, paranoid jealousy, extreme irritability, delusions, and impaired judgment. Other drug abuse may also occur.

C. Growth hormone

1. Growth hormone works by increasing protein production and allows fat to be used for energy rather than muscle glycogen.

2. Side effects of growth hormone include heart disease, impotence, osteoporosis, and death.

D. Androstenedione

1. Androstenedione is a steroid produced naturally in both men and women and is converted in the body to either testosterone or estrogen.

2. Side effects include masculinizing effects in females and feminizing effects in males, premature bone growth cessation, aggression and mood changes, decreased HDL, increased cardiovascular disease, breast cancer, and pancreatic cancer.

3. Androstenedione is banned by the IOC, the NFL, and the NCAA.

E. Caffeine

1. Caffeine makes people feel more alert, full of energy, in a better mood, and more productive.

2. Studies currently contradict each other as to benefits to athletes.

3. Caffeine can cause sleeplessness, anxiety, headache, upset stomach, nervousness, and dehydration. Dehydration can work against athletic performance, since proper water balance is such an important part of nutrition.

4. The IOC has banned caffeine over a certain limit.

F. Creatine monohydrate

1. Creatine is an amino acid, (a protein building block) made in the body by the kidneys and liver. It is found naturally in skeletal muscle. In the body it is converted to phosphocreatine, which serves as a storage reservoir for quick energy.

    2. Side effects include weight gain from excess cellular water, muscle cramping, dehydration, GI stress, nausea, and seizures.

  G. Ephedra

    1. Ephedra is a shrublike plant that is found in desert regions. Ephedra is a stimulant containing the herbal form of ephedrine, an FDA-regulated drug found in over-the-counter asthma medications.

    2. Ephedrine is widely used for weight loss, as an energy booster, and to enhance athletic performance.

    3. Serious adverse effects include hypertension, heart palpitations, neuropathy, myopathy, psychosis, stroke, memory loss, heart rate irregularities, insomnia, nervousness, tremors, seizures, heart attacks, and death.

III. Current IOC, NCAA, and Professional Standards

  A. The International Olympic Committee Medical Commission, in their effort to deal with the problem of doping in the sports world, has established three fundamental principles:

    1. Protection of the health of athletes

    2. Respect for both medical and sports ethics

    3. Equality for all competing athletes

  B. The NCAA has a drug-testing program that mandates urine collection and analysis on specific occasions.

  C. Several professional athletic teams have written policy statements concerning the use of banned substances.

IV. Education for Athletes

  A. Athletes need to understand the inherent dangers and risks associated with the use of dietary supplements and performance enhancers.

  B. The Healthy Competition Foundation is an organization that seeks to educate young people and their families about the potential health dangers of performance-enhancing drugs and to eliminate use of these drugs at all levels of sports.

V. Ethics in Athletics

  A. The athletic code of ethics helps protect and promote the interests of athletics and the coaching profession, primarily to clarify and distinguish ethical practices from those which are detrimental.

  B. Guidelines for players

    1. Players shall represent themselves and their school with honor, proper conduct, and good sportsmanship.

    2. Players shall comply fully with the rulings of officials.

    3. Players shall adhere to the rules of the school and the athletic department.

VOCABULARY REVIEW

Matching

Match the term on the right with the statement on the left. Terms may be used more than once or not at all.

_____ 1. A product intended to enhance the diet

_____ 2. Plant matter used in the form of powders, extracts, teas, and tablets believed to have therapeutic benefits

_____ 3. Often used as a supplement to maintain cartilage in the joints

_____ 4. Often used as a supplement to treat osteoarthritis

_____ 5. Substances used to enhance metabolism and thus work to build up the body tissues

_____ 6. Manmade substances related to the male sex hormones that are used to build muscle and more masculine characteristics

_____ 7. An ergogenic aid produced by the pituitary gland that works to increase amino acid production into protein

_____ 8. A steroid produced in both men and women that can change or enhance the growth and development of masculine or feminine traits

_____ 9. An alkaloid present in coffee, soft drinks, and chocolate that acts as a stimulant

_____ 10. An amino acid found in skeletal muscle stored for quick energy

_____ 11. A substance derived from a shrublike plant used as a stimulant to boost energy and weight loss

_____ 12. A tool used to clarify and distinguish proper practices from those that can be detrimental and harmful

A. anabolic steroids

B. anabolic-androgenic steroids

C. androstenedione

D. athletic code of ethics

E. caffeine

F. chondroitin

G. creatine monohydrate

H. dietary supplement

I. doping

J. ephedra

K. ergogenic aid

L. glucosimine

M. growth hormone

N. medicinal herbs

ACTIVITIES

1. Fat soluble vitamins tend to have toxic effects if taken in excess. Choose one of these vitamins and research just what those toxic effects might be. How much of an excess is needed before these effects become evident?

_____

_____

_____

_____

2. Caffeine is a very common substance in the food and drink people consume. Keep track of your own diet by reading food labels and getting nutrition information. How many sources of caffeine do you use in a given week? Calculate as best you can how much caffeine this represents. Try giving up all of these sources for a month. How are you affected by giving up this stimulant so suddenly?

_____

_____

_____

_____

ONLINE RESEARCH

■ Find cases in the past where athletes have been disqualified from their competition because they were proven to have a banned substance in their system. Describe and report back to the class the circumstances of the case you research.

_____

_____

_____

_____

■ The NFL, NBA, and IOC have testing programs their athletes must take to determine if a banned substance has been used. Major League Baseball, however, has been resistant to developing such a program. Research some of the problems that baseball has dealt with and still faces regarding the use of banned substances, especially steroids, due to the lack of a testing requirement. In your opinion, is it fair to compare a player's performance under the influence of performance enhancers to others, presently and in the past, who have not used such substances?

_____

_____

_____

CHAPTER 10

Sports Psychology

- Sports psychology is a rapidly growing field in which practitioners guide athletes at all levels to find increased success and happiness. Sports psychologists can help athletes set goals, boost self-confidence, stay motivated, enhance self-image, and cope with stress and disappointment.
- Sports psychology is a fast-growing career opportunity. Careers in sports psychology may be pursued in educational, clinical, and research settings.
- Goal setting is one of the most powerful techniques for human motivation. Setting clearly defined goals allows athletes to measure their successes.
- When setting personal goals, keep the following guidelines in mind: express goals positively; set priorities; write down goals; keep operational goals small; set performance goals, not outcome goals; set specific goals; set goals at the right level; set both short-term and long-term goals.
- Imagery allows the individual to practice mentally and prepare for events and eventualities that the athlete can never expect to train for in reality. Simulation attempts to create the circumstances of competition in practice.
- Too much stress can hinder performance and lead to problems in other areas of life. The proper amount of stress, however, can help improve performance.
- Burnout can make an athlete that excels in his or her sport turn away from competition and sports altogether. This can occur due to increased pressure to win, beginning a sport too early, not being involved in other activities, as well as gender differences.

OUTLINE

I. Sports Psychology

   A. Sports psychology is the study of sport and exercise, and the mental (psychological) factors influencing performance. Performance in sport is considered 95% mental, yet most preparation time is devoted to the physical aspects of competition.

   B. Sports psychologists can help athletes develop goals, self-confidence, motivation, positive self-image, and strategies to cope with stress and disappointment.

II. Motivation

A. Motivation serves to activate or energize behavior and give it direction.

B. Extrinsic motivation describes the influence of some type of external reward, such as money or praise.

C. Intrinsic motivation comes from within, such as personal achievement, enjoyment, self-confidence, and positive emotions.

III. Goal Setting

A. Goal setting is one of the most powerful techniques for human motivation, giving both long-term vision and short-term motivation.

B. Setting clearly defined, specific goals allows the individual to achieve more, improve performance, improve the quality of training, increase motivation to achieve at higher levels, increase pride and satisfaction in performance, and improve self-confidence.

C. Other benefits include reduced stress and anxiety, better concentration, more self-confidence, better performance, and more happiness with the performance.

D. To effectively set goals, the athlete should:

1. Express goals positively, taking small steps and celebrating each accomplishment.

2. Set priorities to avoid feeling overwhelmed by too many goals.

3. Write goals down. Written goals help keep the individual from straying off course. The goals should be visible and read each day.

4. Keep operational goals small; otherwise there is a risk of making it appear that progress is not being made.

5. Set performance, not outcome goals. This allows control over achievement of the goals, rather than having outside, uncontrollable influences stand in the way. It is important to assign dates and times for goals so achievement can be measured.

6. Set specific goals.

7. Set goals at the right level. No one will put serious effort into achieving a goal that he or she believes is unrealistic. Setting goals too low can lead to complacency and mediocrity.

8. Goals can be short-term or long-term.

   a. Short-term goals involve time frames of no longer than a few months, perhaps as short as a day.

   b. Long-term goals are set for the distant future. To attain these goals, the athlete must work consistently and reach numerous short-term goals along the way.

IV. Imagery and Simulation

A. Imagery helps create, modify, or strengthen neurologic pathways that are important to the coordination of the muscles. It allows individuals to practice and prepare for events and eventualities that the athlete can never expect to train for in reality.

B. Simulation teaches the brain to cope with circumstances that would not otherwise be encounted until an important competition. It is carried out by making the physical training circumstances as close as possible to the real competition.

V. Strategies to Cope with Stress and Disappointment

A. The proper amount of stress can be healthy and help improve performance. Too much stress can hinder performance and lead to problems in other areas of life.

B. Transitional stress can occur when athletes begin a new sport, go from high school to college, change leagues, change levels of competition, go from junior high to high school, go from college to professional, or retire from athletics.

C. Injury can be devastating to the motivated athlete. Understanding that injuries are part of competitive athletics will allow the athlete to modify goals when injuries do occur.

D. Burnout manifests as dropping out of a sport or quitting an activity that was once enjoyable. This can occur because of frustration due to participating too early in their development, parental pressure of performance and winning, or exhaustion from too much activity.

E. One of the best ways to manage stress is through goal setting. Other ways include meditation, positive thinking, time management, talking to friends, and taking breaks.

VI. Self-Confidence

A. Self-confidence reflects an athlete's assessment of his or her own self-worth.

VII. Career Opportunities

A. Educational sport psychology emphasizes working with athletes in an athletic environment.

B. Clinical sport psychology deals with athletes in a clinical setting.

C. Academic sport psychology focuses on teaching and research.

VOCABULARY REVIEW

Matching

Match the terms on the right with the definitions on the left.

_____ 1. The study of sport and exercise and the psychological factors influencing performance

_____ 2. The process of reviewing and training in the mind only through visualization

_____ 3. Dropping out of a sport or quitting an activity that was once enjoyable

_____ 4. A situation that causes anxiety, focus, or fear

_____ 5. An internal state or condition that serves to activate or energize behavior and give it direction, often based on needs and desires

_____ 6. Identifying clearly defined, specific objectives that are measureable

A. burnout

B. goal setting

C. imagery

D. motivation

E. sports psychology

F. stress

ACTIVITIES

1. Watch a simulated sports psychologist's session with an athlete, either as a live role-play situation or on video. What kinds of questions does the sports psychologist ask? What do you think the purpose of the questions might be? What benefits do you see from these sessions?

_____

_____

_____

_____

_____

2. Describe how you would feel about using such a service for improving your own activities, sports-related or not sports-related.

_____

_____

_____

_____

_____

ONLINE RESEARCH

■ Research the concept of burnout. Look up specific cases referred to on the Internet, and analyze them for what leads to the burnout. Also research how the term _burnout_ applies to other situations and what stresses are put on these people that lead to burnout.

_____

_____

_____

_____

_____

■ Find documented cases on the Internet where sports psychology techniques have led to improvement in performance. Describe what athletes say about the benefits of their participation in psychological procedures.

_____

_____

_____

_____

_____

CHAPTER 11

Assessment and Evaluation
of Sports Injuries

KEY CONCEPTS

■ Assessment and evaluation means compiling subjective and objective data related to the presenting signs and symptoms of a particular injury or disease state. Diagnosis is the ability to take that data and make a scientifically based statement specifying the injury or disease process.

■ The type of injury and the severity of the injury are determined by factors such as anthropomorphic status; mechanism of force, speed, protective equipment in use; and skill level. Anthropomorphic status is based on size, body structure, and maturity level; mechanism of injury is related to the force and energy involved in impact; speed is important because the faster a body is moving, the greater is the force to stop; more force increases the severity of injury; protective equipment, designed to absorb and distribute force, as well as provide added strength to certain areas of the body, avoids or lessens the severity of injury; athletes performing at higher skill levels have a reduced risk of severe injuries, because of their increased knowledge of basic skill sets.

■ Secondary injury surveys provide a thorough, methodical evaluation of an athlete's overall health to reveal additional injuries beyond the initial injury.

■ A systematic approach to injury assessment and evaluation will ensure that no injuries go undiscovered. The approach should be the same each and every time an injury is encountered so that the manner in which the injury is assessed and evaluated becomes routine. First obtain a history; then observe for swelling, deformities, and bleeding; continue by palpating the injury; and finally, perform any special tests to determine the extent of the injury.

■ Having injuries well documented with follow-up care clearly written and followed is essential in the total health of the athlete. There are a wide variety of tools and methods used to document the care the athlete is receiving. The certified athletic trainer determines the tools used in the program.

OUTLINE

I. Assessment and Evaluation of Athletic Injuries

    A. These are important proficiencies that everyone on the athletic health care team must possess.

    B. The knowledge and expertise of the certified athletic trainer, which are applied to evaluate injuries immediately after they occur, helps in getting the proper aid to the athlete as quickly as possible.

        1. Certified athletic trainers can assess and evaluate, but cannot diagnose.

2. Diagnosis is the domain of the licensed health care provider, typically a physician, although sometimes limited by his or her specialty.

3. The certified athletic trainer uses information from the physician to set short- and long-term goals for recovery.

II. Factors Influencing Athletic Injuries

A. Anthropomorphic data include the size, weight, structure, gender, strength, and maturity level of the athletes involved.

B. Mechanism of force comprises all forces involved at the time of an impact, including the direction of the force, its intensity and duration, the activity being undertaken, and the position of the body part at the time of injury.

C. Speed influences the type and severity of athletic injuries because a greater speed of collision causes a greater chance of injury. If athletes of greatly differing skill levels practice together, the lesser skilled athlete typically has the greater chance of being injured.

D. Protective equipment can greatly reduce the risk of injury by absorbing and distributing force that would be otherwise absorbed by the body.

E. The skill level of the athlete influences the rate and severity of athletic injuries because the more skilled athlete has a greater knowledge of what to do to minimize risk of injury.

III. Recognition and Evaluation

A. Recognition of injuries is the process in which the certified athletic trainer determines the probable cause and mechanism of injury, based on direct observation or second hand accounts.

B. The primary injury survey involves controlling life-threatening conditions first and activating the emergency medical services (EMS) when needed. Evaluators look for the basic ABCs.

1. Airway—Open the victim's airway by tilting the head back and lifting the chin, unless spinal injury is suspected, where the jaw-thrust technique is safer.

2. Breathing—Listen, look, and feel for breathing. If the victim is not breathing, give two breaths and check for circulation.

3. Circulation—Check for signs of circulation such as breathing, coughing, or movement in response to the breaths. If there are no signs, start chest compressions.

4. Cardiopulmonary resuscitation (CPR)

a. Only individuals properly trained and certified in CPR should practice this application.

b. The Good Samaritan law protects most helpers from legal actions brought against them, but not if the helper performs procedures for which he or she is not properly trained.

c. For those trained in CPR, the American Heart Association provides guidelines, recommending that rescuers phone 9-1-1 for unresponsive adults before giving CPR, provide one minute of CPR for infants and children to the age of eight before calling 9-1-1, begin chest compressions in the absence of circulation signs, giving about 100 compressions per minute for a person over 8 years old, at a ratio of 15 compressions to 2 breaths. Chest-compression-only CPR is recommended only when the rescuer is unwilling or unable to perform mouth-to-mouth rescue breathing.

C. The secondary injury survey involves the management of nonlife-threatening injuries, entailing a thorough, methodical evaluation of an athlete's overall health. The H.O.P.S. (history, observation, palpation, special tests) evaluation format is often used.

   1. Take your time and be thorough, ruling out the most serious injuries first.

   2. Gather history before touching the athlete. Question others who witnessed the incident.

      a. What happened? Body part injured; description of injury.

      b. When did the injury occur?

      c. What factors influenced the injury? Some factors include position of the body and injured area; activity (collision or contact); speed; direction of force; the force's intensity, duration, and results (twisting, hyperextension, hyperflexion).

      d. Was a sound heard? Was it a pop, snap, rip?

      e. Where is the pain located now? Where was the pain at the time of injury?

      f. Describe the pain: sharp or dull/achy, stabbing, throbbing, constant, cramping, intermittent. Is the pain present at rest or with use of the injured body part? What is its intensity (rate on a scale of 1–10)?

      g. Is neurological function intact? Is there numbness, pins-and-needles prickling, muscle weakness, paralysis, burning sensation?

      h. Is there instability? A sense that something not working right (do not have the person actually use the part in question)

      i. Is there a prior history associated with the injured body part?

   3. Expose the injury to observe the extent of damage. It is important to recognize the privacy of the athlete, exposing the injury in a locker room or private area if at all possible. It is good practice to have a member of the training staff who is the same sex as the injured athlete in attendance for all examinations.

   4. Perform a physical examination

      a. Observation—compare the injured side to the uninjured side, looking especially for deformity, swelling, bleeding, and skin color changes.

      b. Palpation is the touching of the injured athlete, which should be firm enough to cause pain. Palpating too lightly may result in missing a significant injury.

      c. Active motion is movement done by the athlete, asking him or her to move the injured body part through its full range of motion.

      d. Passive motion is movement done by the examiner, with the athlete relaxing all muscles.

      e. Test for strength. Ask the athlete to contract muscles around the injury without moving bones (isometric contraction). Note any visible defects and palpate for knots or lumps in the injured muscle.

      f. Stability tests investigate ligamentous laxity, a stress test for ligaments. A sprain can then be graded I, II, or III. A Grade III sprain or complete tear will require prompt referral to an orthopedic surgeon for repair.

      g. Special tests and examinations, such as the Lachman Anterior Drawer Test for the anterior cruciate ligament, may be necessary to establish the degree of injury.

   5. Functional activity tests determine the level of activity the athlete may resume. Allow the injured athlete to stand, walk, hop, jog, sprint, cut, and twist. Test the uninjured side first for comparison purposes.

6. Sport-specific activity tests determine if the athlete can safely resume the activities of a particular sport. Injured athletes are asked to demonstrate specific maneuvers and actions of their sport, with appropriate supporting devices such as taping.

IV. Return-to-Play Criteria

A. Full strength refers to muscles, ligaments, and tendons being at 100% of pre-injury strength.

B. An athlete must be free from pain during return-to-play performance tests.

C. Skills required for the sport are tested, starting at a low level of intensity and gradually increasing until the athlete is performing at game speed. If at any time the athlete is not able to perform one of the tests, the athlete is not ready to return to the sport.

D. Emotional recovery is just as important as physical recovery. Counseling by the certified athletic trainer or sport psychologist helps the athlete work through any hesitation of returning to play.

V. Documentation of Injuries

A. Advantages of complete documentation

1. One of the biggest reasons for complete documentation is for the follow-up care.

2. Athletes are more likely to get the treatment they need with proper documentation.

3. A profile of injuries in a sport can allow the program director to recognize trends, which can be shared with coaches who can then develop strengthening and stretching programs that may lower injury rates.

4. If a lawsuit is filed for negligence or malpractice, good recordkeeping will help keep the facts straight.

B. SOAP notes refers to a particular format of recording information regarding treatment procedures (subjective, objective, assessment, plan).

1. Subjective is the component that incorporates subjective statements made by the injured athlete, often obtained through history taking.

2. Objective findings include the certified athletic trainer's visual inspection, palpation, and assessment.

3. Assessment of the injury is the certified athletic trainer's professional judgment and impression as to the nature and extent of the injury.

4. Plan includes the first aid treatment rendered to the athlete and the sports therapist's intentions as to disposition, which could include referral for more definitive evaluation or simply application of a splint, wrap, or crutches and a request for reevaluation the next day.

C. The daily sideline injury report is a way to track every athlete who participates in a sport. Data can later be analyzed by computer to reveal injury patterns.

D. The training-room treatment log is filled out by certified athletic trainers as they treat athletes. Everyone taped, wrapped, iced, and so on should be documented.

E. The daily red-cross list can be used to inform coaches of the status of their athletes from one practice to another. After the athlete returns to full practice and competition, his or her name is removed from the list.

F. An athlete medical referral form from the certified athletic trainer taken to the doctor allows accurate communication between the training staff and the physician's office.

VOCABULARY REVIEW

Matching

Match the terms on the right with the statements on the left. Terms may be used once, more than once, or not at all.

_____ 1. The movement done by the athlete to assess injury through range of motion

_____ 2. The act of touching, upon examination, to determine the extent of injury

_____ 3. The level of movement at which the athlete can comfortably work and participate

_____ 4. What a physician believes is wrong, based on skills, expertise, and medical school training

_____ 5. An example of this type of information is an athlete falling three feet above the court to a hardwood floor without a cushioning effect, with the left arm contacting the floor first

_____ 6. Particular types of movement and actions that are related to a particular sport

_____ 7. The movement performed by the examiner while the athlete relaxes all muscles through range of motion

_____ 8. The degree of looseness in the ligaments of a joint

_____ 9. Statistics on size, weight, body structure, gender, strength, and maturity level of a person

_____ 10. All energies involved at the time of impact, including direction, intensity, duration, activity, and position of the body or body part

_____ 11. Basically, this is a stress test for ligaments

_____ 12. What is being tested when a basketball player is asked to sprint, cut, jump, and back peddle

_____ 13. An acronym used to remember the approach to the secondary injury survey

_____ 14. What a certified athletic trainer might think is wrong, based on knowledge and the events that occurred

_____ 15. Includes the basic ABCs in assessing airway, breathing, and circulation

A. anthropomorphic data

B. assessment

C. active motion

D. diagnosis

E. functional activity

F. H.O.P.S.

G. ligamentous laxity

H. mechanism of force

I. palpation

J. passive motion

K. primary injury survey

L. SOAP notes

M. secondary injury survey

N. sport-specific activity

Word Scramble

The scrambled terms describe information that should be gathered first for the secondary injury survey of an athlete's injury. How many can you decipher? (Terms are either one or two words.)

1. aphedhapewtn _____

2. ehwn _____

3. nficiungflostnrcae _____

4. ibyoinodtpos _____

5. vyicatti _____

6. deeps _____

7. froitcdceeiorn _____

8. estyniitn _____

9. snuod _____

10. alnoipinotac _____

11. pihsrpana _____

12. ipnullda _____

13. tntsocna _____

14. ngmpriac _____

15. rtitnmenttie _____

ACTIVITIES

1. Using records of actual injuries that have occurred at your school in the past (names and identifying remarks have been modified or changed to protect privacy), evaluate the information provided as to what use it could be in treating the injured athlete and planning for future rehabilitation. Is there any information missing that might also be helpful?

_____

_____

_____

_____

_____

2. Participate in a role-playing activity, where you are the evaluator of a specific sports injury, and an experienced student trainer plays the part of the injured athlete. Complete the injury evaluation, using forms that are used at your school.

_____

_____

_____

_____

_____

ONLINE RESEARCH

■ Research the kinds of tools physicians use to diagnose sports injuries that are not available to certified athletic trainers. Describe how these devices work, and what information is provided to the physician.

_____

_____

_____

_____

_____

■ Choose three sports, then research the types of injuries that are common and injuries that are unique to those sports. Report your findings back to the class.

_____

_____

_____

_____

_____

CHAPTER 12

Therapeutic Physical Modalities

KEY CONCEPTS

■ Effective application of physical modalities is an important aspect of athletic training and the appropriate care of athletes. Hot and cold treatments, ultrasound, and various electrical modalities can be used to reduce swelling, decrease spasm, and promote healing.

■ Cryotherapy is the use of cooling agents to manage pain and edema and to decrease muscle spasms. Ice packs are effective in the treatment of local areas. The area concerned should be elevated and the cold applied for 15 to 20 minutes. Ice massage is also used for local areas; ice should be rubbed briskly over the injured area for about five minutes. Cold water compression is a technique in which cold water and pressure are simultaneously applied to the injured area. This should be done for 15 to 20 minutes. Ice baths involve immersion of the affected area in a bucket of water with a temperature of 55 to 64 degrees Fahrenheit. Movement exercise can also be done during an ice bath. Hydrocollator packs are used for superficial heating and should be applied for 10 to 20 minutes. Hydrotherapy is a form of superficial heating in which the affected area is immersed in hot, turbulent water for 10 to 20 minutes. Contrast therapy uses alternating cold baths and hot baths for specific time periods.

■ Continuous ultrasound is a form of energy that is transformed into deep heat within the targeted tissue. It facilitates tissue repair in humans.

■ Electrical modalities achieve their effect by stimulating nerve tissue and do not produce heat or cold. These modalities are used to reduce pain and rehabilitate muscles.

OUTLINE

I. Therapeutic Physical Modalities
   A. The therapeutic use of various heating, cooling, and mechanical/electrical modalities used on the human body, including hot and cold treatments, ultrasound, and various electrical modalities.
   B. Modalities are used adjunctively for the management of many sports-related injuries.
   C. Certified athletic trainers decide when a physical modality is warranted and when it is not, and which modality is the correct one to use when necessary.

II. Thermal Modalities

    A. Included are both cryotherapy and the use of heating agents

    B. Cryotherapy

        1. Cold packs, cold bucket baths, and ice massage are all used in the management of pain and edema. They are also effective in decreasing muscle guarding and spasm.

        2. Body reactions to cryotherapy include initial vasoconstriction, reduction of tissue metabolism, decreased nerve conduction velocity, reduction of muscle spasm, secondary vasodilatation, and an increase in muscle strength after treatment.

        3. If left too long, excess blood may be moved to the area by the body.

        4. Cold is the modality of choice for acute injuries, and should be applied as soon as possible, for a maximum of 20 minutes at a time (with two hours before reapplication), three to four times per day.

        5. Ice packs can be made quickly and economically by filling plastic bags with small ice cubes or crushed ice.

            a. Reusable gel packs, which must be stored in the freezer, are appropriate in clinical settings but not too practical for sideline treatments.

            b. Secure the ice pack to the athlete's body by placing it under clothing, wrapped with an elastic bandage or plastic wrap.

            c. It is important to elevate the extremity during ice-pack treatment and limit application to 15 to 20 minutes.

            d. Place a thin cloth barrier between pack and skin.

            e. If the athlete breaks out in a rash with this treatment, discontinue or add more cloth layers between pack and skin.

        6. Ice massage, often used for tennis elbow and shin-splints, involves briskly rubbing ice over the injured area to produce the desired cold effect; the advantage is a shorter treatment of about five minutes.

        7. Cold-water compression, using a commercial sleeve that is filled with ice water and available in different shapes for different body parts, combines the effects of cold with the effects of compression. Therapy time is 15 to 20 minutes.

        8. Ice baths, used for hands or ankles, allows complete, uniform coverage of the area.

            a. Since the body part is not bound to anything, some movement exercises are possible with this therapy.

            b. The ice bath is usually between 55 and 64 degrees Fahrenheit.

            c. Typical therapy time is 10 minutes

        9. Cryotherapy should be used with caution on persons who have thermoregulatory problems, sensory deficits, hypersensitivity to cold, impaired circulation, heart disease, and malignant tissue.

    C. Heating agents

        1. Beneficial effects of heat therapy include reducing pain, promotion of healing, increased range of motion, and muscle relaxation.

        2. Body responses include substantially increased vasodilatation, increased metabolism, capillary pressure and flow, clearance of metabolites, and oxygenation of tissue.

3. Since the body naturally responds with changes similar to the application of heat, heat therapy is usually only appropriate when the natural responses have subsided.

4. Hydrocollator packs are used for superficial heating, are available in many shapes, are easy to apply, and are cost effective.

   a. Once removed from the water, they should be covered with an insulated covering.

   b. Therapy time is 10 to 20 minutes.

   c. Care must be taken to avoid burns, like not trapping the pack and making sure it is comfortably warm, not too hot.

5. Heat is not typically used until 48 to 72 hours after the injury.

6. Heat should not be used with athletes who have impaired circulation, in areas of diminished sensation, when athletes are heat intolerant, or in areas susceptible to bleeding.

7. Hydrotherapy is a form of superficial heating that uses agitated, heated water in a whirlpool, which is typically made of stainless steel or fiberglass and attached to a turbine that mixes air with water under pressure to produce turbulance.

   a. Larger areas can be treated and range-of-motion exercises can be performed.

   b. Disadvantages include the great amount of time needed for filling and cleaning, space for the whirlpool, equipment expense, and the inability to elevate the body part being treated.

   c. Treatment time is 10 to 20 minutes.

8. Contrast therapy uses alternating hot and cold water baths for the ankle, foot, hand, or elbow.

   a. It may be used in the subacute stage of an injury, or 48 to 72 hours after injury to help reduce swelling and pain and increase range of motion.

   b. Contraindications include impaired circulation as a result of diabetes, vascular disease, and a tendency to hemorrhage.

9. Ultrasound (ultrasonic diathermy) is a very high-frequency sound wave that is absorbed by tissues high in protein content, including tendons, ligaments, joint capsules, and muscle tissue. The sound waves are transformed into deep heat within the targeted tissue.

   a. Certified athletic trainers' use of electrical therapeutic modalities is limited by some state practice acts, some states permitting only preparation of the patient, while other states allow a more active role in clinical settings.

   b. Ultrasound should not be used over fluid-filled cavities, eyes, heart, uterus, testes, bone growth plates, fracture sites, artificial joints, and herniated discs. It is also not recommended during the acute stage of an injury.

   c. Treatment is usually 5 to 10 minutes.

III. Therapeutic Electrical Modalities

   A. Physicians and physical therapists are the primary users of therapeutic electrical modalities.

   B. These modalities achieve their effect by stimulating nerve tissue without heat or cold.

C. Electrical Stimulation (E-Stim) Therapy
   1. E-Stim has proven effective in increasing range of motion and muscle strength, reeducation muscle, improving muscle tone, enhancing function, controlling pain, accelerating wound healing, and reducing muscle spasm.
   2. Neuromuscular electrical stimulation (NMES) is the most common type of E-Stim, which stimulates a peripheral nerve to cause either a sensory or a motor response.
   3. Functional electrical stimulation (FES) is the use of E-Stim to improve function.
   4. Transcutaneous electrical nerve stimulation (TENS) is commonly applied with a portable unit for pain control.
   5. Specialized training is a prerequisite for using electrical modalities.
   6. E-Stim should not be used over the carotid sinus, during pregnancy, in individuals with pacemakers, on people who are sensitive to electricity, or any time active motion is contraindicated.

VOCABULARY REVIEW

Matching

Match the terms on the right with the statements on the left. Answers may be used once, more than once, or not at all.

_____ 1. The therapeutic use of cooling agents delivered by several different means

_____ 2. Therapeutic deep heating using high-frequency sound waves; also called ultrasonic diathermy

_____ 3. A technique of cold application used for localized areas

_____ 4. Methods of treatment for injuries

_____ 5. A stainless steel or fiberglass tub with an attached turbine

_____ 6. A form of superficial heating that uses agitated, heated water in a specially designed piece of equipment

_____ 7. The use of electrical impulses to reduce pain by stimulating the sensory and pain-carrying nerves

_____ 8. The use of electrical impulses to produce muscle contractions by stimulating the motor nerves

_____ 9. A stainless steel container filled with hot water used to heat moist packs for superficial heat therapy

A. cryotherapy

B. electrical stimulation (E-Stim)

C. hydrocollator

D. hydrotherapy

E. ice massage

F. modalities

G. transcutaneous electrical nerve stimulation (TENS)

H. ultrasound (US)

I. whirlpool

ACTIVITIES

1. Take a guided tour of your own school's therapeutic modality resources. Write a short paper describing what kinds of treatments described in the textbook athletes can make use of at your school's site. Where in your area do athletes go for the other modalities described in the book?

_____

_____

_____

_____

_____

2. Get trained on how to operate the modalities available to you as a student trainer until you are able to demonstrate the operation yourself.

_____

_____

_____

_____

_____

ONLINE RESEARCH

■ Research different electrical modalities, the historical development of the modality, and its current use. Identify modalities used for treatments in the past that are no longer considered appropriate. Explain what those applications were and why they were finally considered ineffective.

_____

_____

_____

_____

_____

CHAPTER 13

Taping and Wrapping

KEY CONCEPTS

- The primary purpose of taping and wrapping is to provide additional support, stability, and compression for an affected body part. Taping can be used as a preventive measure or as protection for new or healing injuries.
- Supplies needed for taping and wrapping include spray adhesives, underwrap, tape, foam paddings, and tape-removal tools.
- Students should be able to demonstrate basic taping and wrapping techniques described in this chapter.

OUTLINE

I. Taping and Wrapping in the Prevention and Treatment of Athletic Injuries

    A. Taping and wrapping is an important skill for the sports-medicine team.

    B. In can be preventative for athletes who need additional protection or as a treatment for new and healing injuries.

    C. Before tape or wraps are applied, a certified athletic trainer or team physician should complete a full assessment of the athlete's injury.

    D. Athletic tape is hypoallergenic and cotton-backed with adhesive designed to withstand temperature changes.

        1. It should be stored in a cool, relatively dry environment.

        2. Athletic tape is made to be torn easily by holding firmly on each side and pulling at an angle so the force breaks the fibers.

    E. Tape underwrap helps eliminate irritation from repeated taping while providing comfort for the athlete, holding heel and lace pads in place, and keeping tape away from the skin of those athletes allergic to tape.

    F. Spray adherent helps the adhesive tape and underwrap adhere to the skin.

    G. Heel and lace pads help prevent pinching and blistering in friction-prone areas and are used with a lubricant ointment.

    H. Tape-removing tools include specialized scissors and tape-cutting devices designed to slip under the tape and underwrap and quickly slice through the tape without irritation to the athlete.

II. Prophylactic Taping of the Ankle

    A. This is the most common use for athletic tape, adding support and protection from new or additional injury.

    B. Blisters, abrasions, cuts, and athlete's foot must be treated before taping by the certified athletic trainer.

    C. Basic ankle taping

        1. A liberal amount of spray adherent should be used over the entire surface to be taped.

        2. Heel and lace pads are placed in the major friction areas.

        3. Underwrap is applied, maintaining equal tension.

        4. Two anchor strips are applied at the top of the ankle, overlapping half the width of the tape.

        5. Three stirrups are applied around the outside of the ankle.

        6. Two additional stirrups are added.

        7. Cover strips are applied down the ankle.

        8. The bottom of the foot is covered with cover strips.

        9. Two heel locks are applied, which help keep the ankle from moving in either an inverted or everted position.

       10. The final step is called the figure eight.

       11. After taping, gently compress the taped ankle to ensure that the adhesive sticks well.

       12. Be sure to ask the athlete how it feels. A well-taped ankle should show no wrinkles; the taping should be uniform and at the proper tension.

    D. Compression wrap of the ankle

        1. When an athlete sprains an ankle, it will be necessary to control swelling and inflammation with a compression wrap and felt horseshoe.

        2. Elastic wraps should not be applied too tightly (do not stretch more than half of its elastic capability).

        3. Compression wraps can be worn for up to 24 hours, sometimes more.

        4. RICES: rest, ice, compression, elevation, and support are all treatments used for sprained ankles.

III. Low-Dye Taping

    A. Low-dye taping helps to improve foot biomechanics by keeping the athlete from overpronating (foot rotating inward).

    B. If low-dye taping gives significant relief, it is a strong indication that functional orthotics may be appropriate.

    C. This procedure does not always provide relief. If there is no relief after two to three procedures, low-dye taping should be discontinued.

IV. Turf-Toe Taping

    A. Turf toe, technically called a metatarsalphalangeal joint (MPJ) sprain, can occur after a forceful hyperextension (upward bending) of the big toe, causing damage to the ligaments and joint capsule.

    B. Taping can help stabilize the MPJ of the big toe, keeping it from hyperextending.

V. Achilles-Tendon Taping

    A. The Achilles tendon is the largest tendon in the body, joining the lower leg gastrocnemius and soleus muscles to the heel bone (calcaneus).

B. Most ruptures of the Achilles tendon occur with the contraction of the calf muscles.

C. Taping is an effective way to relieve strain and overstretching.

VI. Shin-Splint Taping

A. Shin splints, or medial tibial stress syndrome (MTSS), should be properly diagnosed prior to treatment.

B. Circumferential elastic taping is a common method for providing some relief, giving gentle compression that relieves some of the discomfort of MTSS.

VII. Wrist taping adds support to the wrist above and beyond the wrist support products available commercially.

VIII. Thumb Taping

A. For a mild sprain, proper taping allows safe return to play.

B. A simple method to keep the thumb from hyperextending is to tape the thumb to the adjacent finger, maintaining the normal spacing between the two.

IX. Finger support can be obtained from a simple buddy taping procedure.

X. Elbow Taping

A. Hyperextension of the elbow is normally the result of falling on an outstretched arm or hand.

B. Taping will prevent hyperextension and prevent hypermobility (a body part moving beyond its normal range of motion).

XI. Groin wrap, uses a specialized wrap designed for this area to help with rehabilitation and recovery.

XII. Hip flexor wrap is identical to groin wrap, except that it goes in the opposite direction.

XIII. Thigh compression wrap can help control the extent of bleeding within the muscle, common when the athlete receives a severe blow to the thigh.

VOCABULARY REVIEW

Matching

Match the terms on the right with the statements on the left. Terms may be used once, more than once, or not at all.

_____ 1. A lightweight foam material used as a base to apply tape over; this helps reduce irritation caused by the tape

_____ 2. Reduced potential for causing an allergic reaction

_____ 3. The process of taping around an extremity or body part

_____ 4. An aerosol liquid that provides a tacky surface to help the underwrap and tape stay in place

_____ 5. The ability of a body part to move beyond the normal range of motion

_____ 6. Any agent that provides preventative measures or guards against injury

A. circumferential

B. hypoallergenic

C. hypermobility

D. prophylactic

E. spray adherent

F. underwrap

ACTIVITY

1. The most important activity in this chapter, like the textbook says, is to practice, practice, then practice some more with the taping procedures described in the textbook. Expect to demonstrate these procedures more than once, from now until the end of the course.

_____

_____

_____

_____

_____

ONLINE RESEARCH

■ Choose one method of taping, then search the Internet for alternative ways to achieve the same goal by taping and wrapping.

_____

_____

_____

_____

_____

CHAPTER 14

Kinesiology

KEY CONCEPTS

- The study of kinesiology focuses on exercise stress, movement efficiency, and fitness.

- The articular system is a series of joints that allows movement of the human body.

- The three classifications of joints are synarthroses, amphiarthroses, and diarthroses. The synarthric joints are immovable. The amphiarthric joints are slightly movable. The diarthric joints are freely movable. Most joints in the human body are diarthric joints.

- There are six types of diathroses (synovial joints) pivot joint, gliding joint, hinge joint, condyloid or ellipsoidal joint, ball-and-socket joint, and saddle joint. Each type of joint allows a particular type of motion.

- The different types of movement in synovial joints are flexion, which decreases the angle between bones; extension, which increases the angle between two bones; hyperextension, which is the ability to move beyond the normal range; abduction which is moving the limbs away from the midline of the body; adduction, which is moving the limbs toward the midline; rotation, turning the bone on its axis; circumduction, rotating the distal end of a limb with the proximal end stationary; supination, moving the forearm so that it is anterior or superior; pronation, moving the forearm so it is posterior or inferior; plantar flexion, which extends the foot with toes pointing down; dorsiflexion, which brings the toes upward toward the lower leg; inversion, turning the sole of the foot medially; eversion, turning the sole laterally; protraction, moving the bone forward; retraction, moving the bone backward; elevation, which is lifting the bone superiorly; depression, moving the bone inferiorly; and opposition, moving the thumb to touch the finger tips.

- In medicine, professionals refer to sections of the body in terms of anatomical planes or flat surfaces. The coronal plane allows discussion of anatomy related to the front or back of the body. The sagittal plane allows discussion of anatomy related to the right and left halves of the body. The axial plane allows discussion related to the upper or lower portion of the body.

- Closed- and open-chain exercises provide different benefits. Closed-chain exercises emphasize compression of joints, whereas open-chain exercises involve shearing forces. Open-chain exercises do not provide as much stability as closed-chain exercises.

OUTLINE

I. Kinesiology

    A. Kinesiology is a multidisciplinary study focusing on exercise stress, movement efficiency, and fitness.

    B. The articular system is a series of joints that allows movement of the human body.

    C. Where two bones come into contact, a joint articulation is formed, which may be immovable, slightly moveable, or freely movable. Arthrology is the study of joint structure and function.

II. Classification of Joints

    A. Synarthroses are joints that lack a synovial cavity and are held closely together by fibrous connective tissue. They are immovable.

        1. Sutures are the joints between skull bones, separated by a thin layer of dense fibrous connective tissue. They begin to fuse together shortly after birth. Once fused, the joints are immovable.

        2. Syndesmoses joints are connected by ligaments and are very slightly moveable; sometimes classified as an amphiarthrosis joint.

        3. A gomphosis is a joint in which a conical process fits into a socket and is held there by ligaments, like teeth held to the jaw bones.

    B. Amphiarthroses are slightly movable joints connected by hyaline cartilage or fibrocartilage.

    C. Diarthroses (synovial joints) are freely movable, with bone ends covered with articular cartilage, and separated by a space called the joint cavity.

        1. Within the joint is a joint capsule; its outer layer is made of ligaments and inner synovial membrane secretes synovial fluid for lubrication.

        2. Pivot joints allow a bone to move around a central axis, creating rotational motion, as in the joint between the atlas and axis of the vertebral column.

        3. Gliding joints allow movement in a sliding motion, as between carpals of the wrist and tarsals of the foot.

        4. Hinge joints allow only flexion and extension, as in the two distal joints of the fingers.

        5. Condyloid or ellipsoidal joints can move in many directions, but cannot rotate, as in the joint between the metacarpals and phalanges of the hand or metatarsals and phalanges of the foot.

        6. Ball-and-socket joints include those in which one bone's rounded end fits into a concave cavity on another bone, providing the widest range of movement possible in joints, as in the femur's connection to the hip bones, or the humerus and the bones of the pectoral girdle.

        7. The saddle joint occurs in the thumb, where the two bones have both concave and convex regions, and allows the thumb to touch each of the fingertips, plus many other movements.

III. Movements of Diarthroses (Synovial Joints)

    A. The stability of a joint is determined by the shape of the bones at the joints, the ligaments that join the bones, and muscle tone, which is usually the main stabilizing factor.

   B. Flexion is a movement that decreases the angle between the bones.

   C. Extension is the act of increasing the angle between the bones.

   D. Hyperextension is the ability to move beyond the normal range of motion.

   E. Abduction describes limbs that move away from the body's midline.

   F. Adduction describes limbs that move toward the midline.

   G. Rotation is the turning of a bone around its axis toward or away from the midline.

   H. Circumduction is when the proximal end of a limb remains stationary and the distal point moves in a circle.

   I. Supination describes moving the forearm so that it is anterior or superior

   J. Pronation is moving the forearm so that it is posterior or inferior.

   K. Plantar flexion is a movement that extends the foot with the toes pointing down.

   L. Dorsiflexion involves flexing the foot so the toes move toward the lower leg.

   M. Inversion turns the sole of the foot medially (inward).

   N. Eversion turns the sole of the foot laterally (outward).

   O. Protraction involves moving a bone forward in a transverse plane.

   P. Retraction involves moving a bone backward in a transverse plane.

   Q. Elevation moves a bone superiorly along a frontal plane.

   R. Depression moves a bone inferiorly along a frontal plane.

   S. Opposition involves moving the thumb to touch the fingertips.

IV. Anatomical Planes

   A. The anatomical position refers to a person standing erect, eyes forward, arms at the side, palms and toes facing forward.

   B. The coronal, or frontal plane, is a vertical plane running from side to side, dividing the body into anterior (front) and posterior (back) portions.

   C. The sagittal, or lateral, plane is a vertical plane running from front to back, dividing the body into left and right portions.

   D. The axial, or transverse, plane is a horizontal plane that divides the body into an upper and lower portion.

V. Open and Closed Kinematic Chains

   A. In a closed kinematic chain exercise, the end of the chain farthest from the body is in a fixed position.

     1. Examples include squats, push-ups, or pull-ups.

     2. These movements emphasize compression of joints, making the joint more stable.

     3. More muscles and joints get involved, leading to better coordination around each structure.

   B. In open kinematic chain exercises, the body part farthest from the body moves the most.

     1. Examples include seated leg extensions and kicking a ball.

     2. These movements involve more shearing force parallel to the joint, making the joint less stable.

VOCABULARY REVIEW

Matching

Match the terms on the right with the statements on the left. Terms may be used once, more than once, or not at all.

_____ 1. A freely movable joint that allows bones to move about one another in many different directions, but cannot rotate

_____ 2. An inflammation of the entire joint

_____ 3. An inflammation of the synovial cavity, caused by excess stress or tension

_____ 4. Movement allowing the proximal end of the limb to remain stationary while the distal end moves in a circle

_____ 5. The body part in a sequence of body parts farthest from the trunk is fixed during movement

_____ 6. Movement of a bone downward in a frontal plane

_____ 7. Freely movable joints; also know as synovial joints

_____ 8. The connecting point of two bones

_____ 9. The body part in a sequence of body parts farthest from the trunk is free during movement

_____ 10. Movement allowing the foot to flex

_____ 11. Movement of a bone upward in a frontal plane

_____ 12. Movement of the sole of the foot outward

_____ 13. Movement allowing limbs to move away from the midline of the body

_____ 14. Movement allowing the limbs to move toward the midline of the body

_____ 15. Slightly moveable joints where bones are connected by hyaline cartilage or fibrocartilage

_____ 16. Movement that allows the angle between two bones to increase

_____ 17. Movement that allows the angle between two bones to decrease

_____ 18. A joint that allows bones to move in a sliding motion

A. abduction
B. adduction
C. amphiarthroses
D. arthritis
E. arthrology
F. articular cartilage
G. axial plane
H. ball-and-socket joint
I. bursitis
J. circumduction
K. closed kinematic chain
L. concave
M. condyloid (ellipsoidal) joint
N. convex
O. depression
P. diarthroses
Q. dorsiflexion
R. elevation
S. eversion
T. extension
U. flexion
V. gliding joints
W. gomphosis
X. gout
Y. inversion
Z. joint articulation
AA. open kinematic chain
BB. opposition
CC. plantar flexion
DD. pronation
EE. retraction
FF. rheumatoid arthritis
GG. rotation
HH. saddle joint
II. sagittal plane
JJ. supination
KK. sutures
LL. synarthroses
MM. syndesmoses
NN. synovial fluid
OO. synovial joint
PP. synovial membrane

_____ 19. An immovable joint in which a conical process fits into a socket held in place by ligaments

_____ 20. The study of joints

_____ 21. Movement of the radius and ulna anterior or superior

_____ 22. An immovable, fused joint found only in the skull and separated by a layer of dense fibrous connective tissue that unites the bones of the skull

_____ 23. Connective tissue covering the ends of long bones

_____ 24. A connective tissue disorder resulting in severe inflammation of small joints

_____ 25. Movement of a bone around an axis toward or away from the body

_____ 26. A horizontal, flat surface dividing the body into upper and lower parts

_____ 27. A joint allows movement in almost any direction, providing the widest range of movement possible among all joint types

_____ 28. An accumulation of uric acid crystals in the joint at the base of the large toe and other joints of the foot

_____ 29. Movement allowing the foot to extend

_____ 30. Movement of the sole of the foot inward

_____ 31. Movement of the thumb to touch each finger

_____ 32. A lubricating substance found in joint cavities

_____ 33. A half-circle-shaped indentation on a surface

_____ 34. A double layer of connective tissue that lines joint cavities and produces synovial fluid

_____ 35. Movement of the radius or ulna posterior or inferior

_____ 36. Movement of a bone backward in a transverse plane

_____ 37. A joint that occurs when two bones have both concave and convex regions with the shapes of the bones complementing one another and allowing a wide range of movement.

_____ 38. A vertical, flat surface running from front to back

_____ 39. A half-circle-shaped protrusion on a surface

_____ 40. Freely movable joint; also known as a diarthrosis

_____ 41. Immovable joints that lack a synovial cavity and are held together by fibrous connective tissue

_____ 42. Joints where the bones are connected by ligaments

Crossword Puzzle

Identify the terms described in the puzzle clues, then write the letters in the boxes. (Many terms are more than one word.)

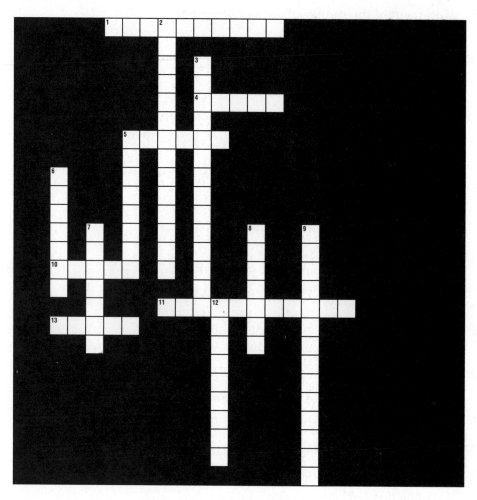

Across

1. inflammation of fibrous connective tissue in a joint _____
4. a joint allowing rotational movement _____
5. an immovable joint in the skull _____
10. a plane dividing the body into upper and lower parts _____
11. study of physical activity and movement _____
13. a joint that only allows flexion and extension _____

Down

2. a bacterial infection that can be carried by blood to the joints _____
3. movement beyond the natural range of motion _____
5. a type of fluid that lubricates joint movement _____
6. a plane that is vertical, running from side to side _____
7. a joint that allows bones to move in a sliding motion _____
8. the angle between bones decreases _____
9. a degenerative joint disease _____
12. movement of a bone upward in a frontal plane _____

ACTIVITIES

1. Practice demonstrating the 18 different synovial joint movements until you are ready to perform them in a testing situation, where the tester tells you a movement, such as saying the word "dorsiflexion" and you demonstrate that movement without the use of any references to textbook, notes, or any other source.

_____

_____

_____

_____

_____

2. On a human skeleton and with your own body, demonstrate examples of each type of joint and how each joint can move.

_____

_____

_____

_____

_____

ONLINE RESEARCH

■ Choose a joint disorder or injury and research current information about its cause and treatment, including details not mentioned in the textbook. Then write a paper explaining what you have found.

_____

_____

_____

_____

CHAPTER 15

Bleeding and Shock

KEY CONCEPTS

- The cardiorespiratory system is the body system responsible for providing oxygen and nutrients to all of the body's cells, as well as ridding the body of the waste products of metabolism.

- Components of the circulatory system include the heart, arteries, arterioles, capillaries, venules, and veins.

- The right side of the heart pumps blood through the lungs, where the blood picks up oxygen to be delivered to the cells of the body. The left side of the heart pumps blood to all other parts of the body, delivering oxygen-rich blood to the cells and picking up waste products to be delivered to the lungs and kidneys for removal.

- Blood pressure pushes the blood through the arteries of the body and is provided by the contraction of the left ventricle and the recoil of elastic artery walls. The systolic pressure is the larger of the two numbers used to represent blood pressure and occurs when the left ventricle contracts. The diastolic pressure is the lower of the two numbers and occurs when the left ventricle relaxes. The pressure results from the recoil of elastic artery walls. Pulse is the expansion and recoil of elastic artery walls as the blood passes through them, which can be felt at certain locations where the arteries are close to the body's surface.

- Standard precautions were developed to prevent contact with the blood of patients who may have infections that can be spread through bodily fluids and blood. All patients should be assumed to be infectious for bloodborne diseases.

- Arterial, venous, and capillary bleeding differ from each other: arterial bleeding occurs in great amounts in a pulsating fashion; venous bleeding is a slower, nonpulsating bleeding; capillary bleeding is more of an oozing than a flow of blood.

- Shock is a precursor to death. When the body is in a shock state, certain areas are deprived of oxygen. This could result in damage to those parts of the body, and, if prolonged and untreated, could result in death.

OUTLINE

I. The Cardiorespiratory System

    A. The cardiorespiratory system includes the functions of the heart, blood vessels, circulation, and gas exchange between the blood and the atmosphere.

    B. Within the lungs, blood is enriched with oxygen and releases carbon dioxide, referred to as respiration.

II. The Circulatory System

    A. The circulatory system involves the heart, arteries, capillaries, and veins as blood circulates throughout the body, transporting nutrients, wastes, and gases from one location to another.

    B. The heart is really two pumps incorporated into a single organ.

        1. The right side of the heart pumps blood to the lungs and back to the heart's left side, referred to as the pulmonary circulation.

        2. The left side of the heart pumps blood to the rest of the body and back to the heart's right side, referred to as the systemic circulation.

        3. Each side of the heart consists of an atrium and a ventricle. The two sides are separated by a wall called a septum (more specifically, the interatrial septum and the interventricular septum).

        4. Valves between the atria and ventricles keep blood flowing in one direction, from atrium to ventricle.

            a. The mitral (bicuspid) valve separates the left atrium from the left ventricle.

            b. The tricuspid valve separates the right atrium from the right ventricle.

        5. Blood enters the right atrium of the heart through the superior vena cava and the inferior vena cava, and blood leaves the right ventricle through the pulmonary artery, which leads to the lungs.

        6. Blood enters the left atrium (from the lungs) through the pulmonary veins, and blood leaves the left ventricle through the aorta, the largest artery in the body.

    C. Blood is composed of many different parts with many different functions.

        1. Platelets are fragments of a very large cell, the megakaryocyte. Platelets have the ability to stick together and function in the first stages of blood clotting.

        2. Plasma is the liquid portion of the blood that carries blood cell, dissolved nutrients, waste products, antibodies, clotting proteins, chemical messengers such as hormones, and proteins.

        3. Red blood cells are the most numerous of the blood cell types. They no longer possess a nucleus, but are very specialized carriers of oxygen attached to a molecule called hemoglobin, which is responsible for the red color of red blood cells and blood.

        4. There are five different types of white blood cells. All have the ability to recognize and destroy invading organisms.

    D. Blood vessels

        1. Arteries are blood vessels that carry blood away from the heart. Arteries continue to branch into smaller vessels the further they get from the heart. The smallest arteries are called arterioles.

2. Veins are blood vessels that carry blood toward the heart. Blood starts in the smallest veins, called venules, that combine with larger and larger veins until they reach the heart. Many veins have internal one-way valves that keep the blood flowing in the right direction, helped along by the contraction of skeletal muscles near the veins.

3. Capillaries connect arteries to veins. It is through the very thin capillary walls that oxygen and carbon dioxide are exchanged, and nutrients and wastes are exchanged.

E. Coronary arteries provide circulating blood to the tissues of the heart, which requires large amounts of oxygen and nutrients to continue its contractions.

III. The Heart's Conduction System

A. The heart's conduction system is made of specialized cells within the heart that coordinate the beating of the heart by the way they conduct electrical signals.

B. The cardiac conduction system keeps the two atria contracting together, followed by the two ventricles contracting together.

IV. Blood Pressure

A. Blood pressure is represented by two numbers: the systolic and diastolic.

1. The systolic pressure is the highest pressure number and corresponds to the contraction of the left ventricle.

2. The diastolic pressure is the lower pressure number and occurs when the ventricle relaxes. It is due to recoil of the elastic arterial walls.

3. The average adult blood pressure is 120 mm/Hg (millimeters of mercury) for the systolic and 80 mm/Hg for the diastolic, recorded as 120/80. The pulse pressure is the difference between systolic and diastolic, which in the average case, would be 40.

B. Athletes often have much lower than average blood pressures, due to the heart being stronger and more efficient.

C. Pulse is created by alternate expansion and contraction of the arteries as blood flows through them. Pulse can be felt in seven different arteries of the body.

1. Brachial artery—located at the crook of the elbow, along the inner border of the biceps muscle

2. Common carotid artery—in the neck, along the front margin of the sternocleidomastoid muscle, near the lower edge of the thyroid cartilage

3. Femoral artery—in the groin (inguinal) area

4. Dorsalis pedis artery—on the anterior surface of the foot, below the ankle joint

5. Popliteal artery—behind the knee

6. Radial artery—at the wrist, on the same side as the thumb

7. Temporal artery—slightly above the outer edge of the eye

D. The pulse rate for athletes is also significantly lower than the average.

E. The target heart rate is expressed as a range of percentages of the maximum heart rate (max. heart rate = 220 – age) that is safe to reach during exercise.

1. For most people, the American Heart Association recommends an exercise target heart rate ranging from 50% to 75% of the maximum heart rate.

2. Maintaining the target heart rate for a period of 15 to 20 minutes each day will produce health benefits.

V. Body Substance Isolation

    A. Gloves must be worn when treating any injury involving body fluids, especially blood.

        1. Sterile gloves made of latex have outstanding barrier properties and are excellent for protecting both health care workers and patients.

        2. Nonlatex synthetic gloves are available for those people with latex allergies.

        3. Gloves must be discarded properly (in a garbage can lined with a red biohazard bag) so that secondary exposure does not occur.

    B. Eyewear must meet the following minimum requirements:

        1. Provide adequate protection against the hazards for which they are designed

        2. Be reasonably comfortable

        3. Fit securely, without interfering with movement or vision

        4. Be capable of being disinfected if necessary, and be easy to clean

        5. Fit over, or incorporate prescription eyewear

    C. Surgical masks should be worn if there is a danger of infectious disease spreading from the athlete to the training staff.

VI. OSHA Guidelines for Infectious Disease Control

    A. Standard precautions are infection control guidelines designed to protect workers from exposure to diseases spread by blood and certain body fluids. All patients should be assumed to be infectious for bloodborne diseases such as AIDS and hepatitis B.

    B. Guidelines include:

        1. Wash hands before and after all patient or specimen contact.

        2. Treat the blood of all patients as potentially infectious.

        3. Treat all linen soiled with blood or body secretions as potentially infectious.

        4. Wear gloves if contact with blood or body fluids is possible.

        5. Immediately place used syringes in a nearby impermeable sharps container; do not recap or manipulate the needles or sharps in any way.

        6. Wear protective eyewear and a mask if splatter with blood or body fluids is possible.

        7. Wear a mask if there is a risk of infection by TB or other airborne organisms.

VII. Wound Care

    A. Anyone giving aid to an injured athlete must first protect himself or herself from contamination and the risk of injury.

    B. Irrigate the wound with clean, cool water to wash away any foreign particles in the wound itself. If this is not possible, physician referral is necessary.

    C. Minor cuts and abrasions should be washed, dried with a sterile gauze sponge, and treated with first aid cream to prevent infection. Then apply a sterile bandage, which should be replaced daily, more often if it gets wet or soaked through with drainage.

    D. Bandages and dressings will ensure proper healing and infection control. The material must be large enough to cover the injury.

        1. The gauze dressing is made of cotton, woven into a flexible and absorbent cloth.

        2. The occlusive dressing is designed to prevent air and moisture from entering or escaping the wound. They are often impregnated with a petroleum gel or covered with a thin plastic film.

    3. Bandage guidelines:

       a. Select the proper size and material for the injury.

       b. Remove anything that interferes with bandaging, such as rings, watches, earrings, and bracelets.

       c. Never reuse a dressing or bandage. Only use sterile material.

       d. The bandage should be snug, but not too tight.

       e. Leave fingers and toes exposed (if possible) so that circulation can be checked.

VIII. Bleeding

    A. Arterial bleeding can be severe. A cut artery issues bright red blood that spurts or pulses corresponding to the heart beat.

    B. Venous bleeding is steady, and the blood will appear bluish-red because of lower oxygen levels.

       1. Veins are closer than arteries to the surface; therefore, it is easier to control venous bleeding.

       2. Direct pressure and compression bandaging are effective ways to manage venous bleeding. Additional layers of dressing may be needed. A physician should be seen immediately.

    C. Capillary bleeding is slow and typically oozes. Blood clotting normally occurs rapidly.

       1. Slow bleeding does carry a greater risk of infection.

       2. Bandage with a sterile dressing.

IX. Shock

    A. Shock is a precursor of death. Prompt recognition, treatment, and control of shock are crucial for the survival of the victim.

       1. Shock occurs when the circulatory system fails to send blood to all parts of the body.

       2. The result is damage to parts of the body such as the limbs, lungs, heart, and brain.

    B. Hemorrhagic shock is the loss of blood from an injury, internal or external.

    C. Respiratory shock occurs when the lungs are unable to supply enough oxygen to the blood, caused by disease, illness, or pulmonary contusion (bruising of the lungs).

    D. Neurogenic shock is the loss of vascular control by the nervous system.

    E. Cardiogenic shock is caused by inadequate functioning of the heart.

    F. Metabolic shock occurs when there is a severe loss of body fluids.

    G. Anaphylactic shock is caused by a severe allergic reaction.

    H. Septic shock is a life-threatening reaction to a severe infection.

    I. Psychogenic shock is a physiological response to fear, stress, or emotional crisis, and causes a person to faint.

    J. Signs and symptoms of shock include:

       1. Restlessness and anxiety

       2. Weak and rapid pulse

       3. Cold and clammy skin

       4. Profuse sweating

       5. Face that becomes pale and may eventually become cyanotic (blue) around the mouth

6. Shallow respirations

7. Thirst

8. Nausea and vomiting

9. Blood pressure that drops slowly and steadily

10. Loss of consciousness

K. Shock may not cause all of the signs. If a person has been seriously injured, the onset of shock should always be suspected. Treat for shock before it happens.

L. General care and treatment for shock include the following:

1. Maintain a clear airway so breathing is not impaired.

2. Control all bleeding.

3. Elevate extremities 12 inches to help control swelling.

4. Splint fractures and elevate if well stabilized.

5. Avoid rough and excessive handling that may cause additional injury.

6. Prevent loss of body heat. If possible, a blanket should be placed under the victim as well as on top.

7. In general, keep the victim in a supine position. A person complaining of chest pain may be more comfortable in a semi-reclining position.

8. Do not give the victim anything to eat or drink to avoid choking or vomiting.

9. Record vital signs (pulse, blood pressure, respiration rate) every five minutes. This will give EMS personnel important data.

10. Constantly reassure the victim, keeping him or her calm.

11. Activate EMS. Call 911 immediately.

VOCABULARY REVIEW

Matching

Match the terms on the right with the definitions on the left. Terms may be used once, more than once, or not at all.

_____ 1. The nervelike cells within the heart muscle that coordinate the contractions of the heart so that the atria contract first, followed by the ventricles

_____ 2. The largest artery in the body; it receives blood from the left ventricle of the heart

_____ 3. A petroleum-based dressing with a thin, plastic film designed to keep out air and moisture from a wound

_____ 4. The yellowish liquid of the blood

_____ 5. The upper chambers of the heart

_____ 6. Arteries that bring nutrients and oxygen to the muscle tissues of the heart

_____ 7. The lower number in a blood pressure reading, representing the pressure that is maintained by the recoil of elastic artery walls after they are expanded by the contraction of the left ventricle

_____ 8. A serious condition of the body that is the precursor to death

_____ 9. The lower chambers of the heart

_____ 10. A woven, flexible, absorbent cloth applied to a wound

_____ 11. Tiny cell fragments in blood that aid in clotting

_____ 12. The smallest veins

_____ 13. The higher number in a blood pressure reading, representing the pressure that is created by the contraction of the left ventricle

_____ 14. An artery leaving the right ventricle that brings blood with low oxygen levels and high carbon dioxide levels to the lungs for gas exchange

_____ 15. The structures of the body involved in gas exchange and gas transport; it includes structures of the circulatory system and the respiratory system

A. aorta

B. arteries

C. arterioles

D. atria

E. capillaries

F. cardiac conduction system

G. cardiorespiratory system

H. coronary arteries

I. diastolic

J. gauze dressing

K. occlusive dressing

L. plasma

M. platelets

N. pulmonary artery

O. pulse

P. pulse pressure

Q. septum

R. shock

S. systolic

T. target heart rate

U. standard precautions

V. veins

W. ventricles

X. venules

_____ 16. Blood vessels that carry blood from the heart to all organs and cells in the body

_____ 17. The difference between the diastolic and systolic pressures in the heart

_____ 18. The muscular wall that separates the atria and the ventricles

_____ 19. The percentage of the maximum heart rate that is safe to reach during exercise; it is typically 50% to 75% of maximum

_____ 20. Infection control guidelines designed to protect workers from exposure to disease, spread by contact with blood or other bodily fluids

_____ 21. Blood vessels that carry blood toward the heart from all organs and cells in the body

_____ 22. The smallest blood vessels with walls; so thin that exchange of gases, nutrients, and waste products occurs easily

_____ 23. The smallest arteries

_____ 24. The rhythmical beating of the heart

ANATOMY IDENTIFICATION

1. Label and color the structures of the heart.

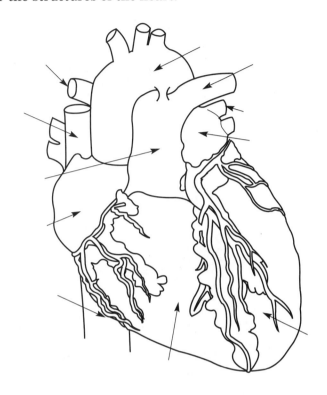

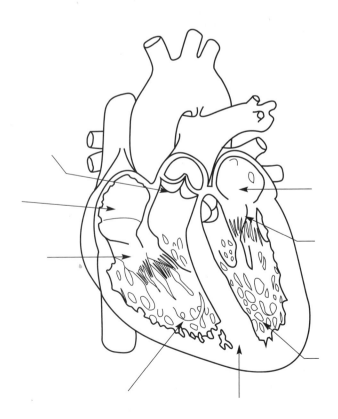

2. Label and color the arteries (below) and the veins (on page 101).

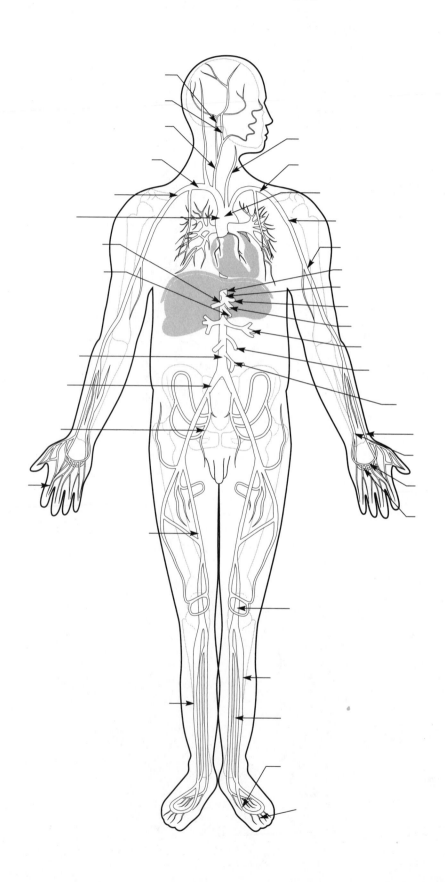

2. (continued)

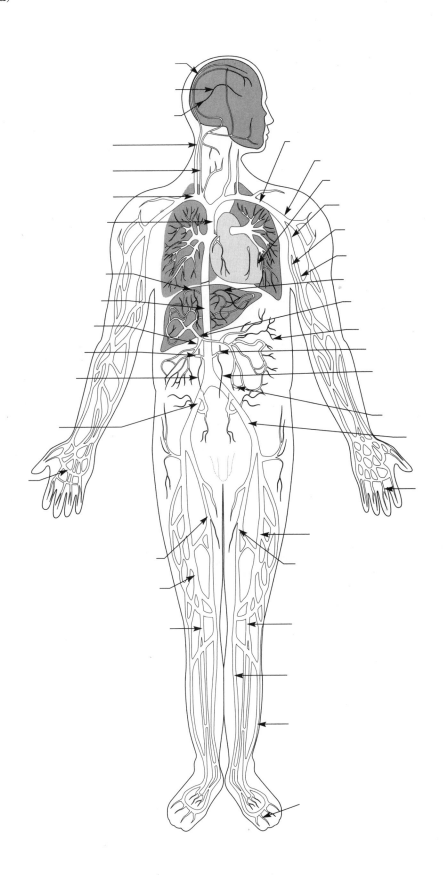

3. Label and color the parts of the capillary bed.

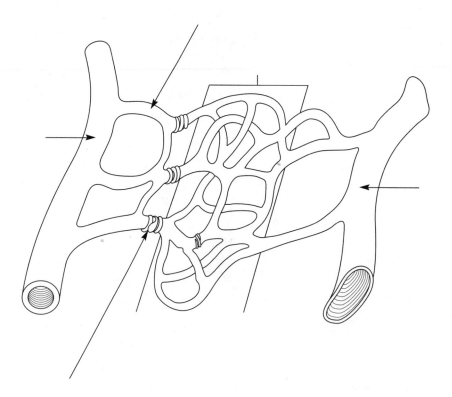

ACTIVITIES

1. Get a manual sphygmomanometer and stethoscope, and practice taking the blood pressure of other students in the classroom. Write a paper on blood pressure, describing exactly what is heard through the stethoscope and why it sounds as it does. Take your blood pressure every day for a week or two, and then graph your results and calculate an average. How does your average compare to the average blood pressure for your age and sex?

   _____

   _____

   _____

   _____

   _____

2. Using a stethoscope, listen to your heartbeat and/or another student's heartbeat. Describe what you hear. What is happening in the heart that gives the sound that you hear?

   _____

   _____

   _____

   _____

   _____

3. On another student in the classroom, locate two pulse points, one close to the heart and one far from the heart. How much delay is there between the two pulses for each heartbeat? Describe why this delay exists.

   _____

   _____

   _____

   _____

   _____

ONLINE RESEARCH

■ Research what a heart murmur is and how this condition is dealt with today.

   _____

   _____

   _____

   _____

■ Low blood pressure in athletes is a normal condition of their heart being stronger and more efficient. Research conditions on the Internet that also show low blood pressure, but are not signs of a healthy heart

_____

_____

_____

_____

_____

CHAPTER 16

The Bones and Soft Tissues

KEY CONCEPTS

- The skeleton has two main parts: the axial skeleton and the appendicular skeleton. The axial skeleton consists of the skull, spine, ribs, and sternum. The appendicular skeleton consists of the shoulder and pelvic girdles and the attached limb bones.

- The functions of the skeletal system are to aid in movement of the body; support and protect internal body organs; produce red and white blood cells; and provide a storehouse for minerals.

- Fractures can be classified by the degree of injury to the bone. There are six types. The simple fracture is a break in the bone that does not penetrate the skin; the compound fracture is a break in the bone that penetrates the skin; the greenstick fracture is an incomplete break; the stress fracture is the result of overuse or weakness; and the epiphyseal plate fracture is a break that occurs at or near the growth plate.

- There are three main types of muscle: skeletal muscle, which is under voluntary control and aids in movement; smooth muscle, which is not under voluntary control but is controlled by the central nervous system; and cardiac muscle, which is involuntary and makes up the heart.

- A strain is the result of twisting or pulling a muscle or tendon. It is characterized by pain, muscle spasm, and muscle weakness. Signs of a strain may include localized swelling, cramping, inflammation, and some loss of muscle function.

- The function of nerve cells is to carry impulses by creating electrical charges. This is done by moving electrically charged ions across a membrane. Ions move from an area of higher concentration to an area of lower concentration.

- A nerve injury occurs because of pressure, stretching, or cutting of the nerve. Damage to a nerve interrupts the nerve's signals to the brain and can impair motor function and sensation as a result. Treatment for a cut nerve is to sew together the myelin sheath around both ends of the nerve. The goal is to save the cover so that new nerve fibers can grow.

- The treatments for soft-tissue injuries vary by injury: abrasions are treated by washing with soap and water, applying antibiotic ointment, and leaving them open to air if not bleeding or oozing; lacerations are treated by cleaning them with soap and water and applying a bandage with pressure to stop the bleeding; avulsions must be cleaned and any remaining flap of skin should be replaced in its original position (completely detached skin can be placed on ice), often

(continues)

(continued)

followed up with treatment by a doctor; puncture wounds should be examined to determine if the object is still in the wound, if underlying structures are damaged, and if the object was contaminated and could increase the risk of infection, then checked by a physician; contusions can be treated with ice, compressive dressings, and anti-inflammatory medications; hematomas are treated with compression, cold packs, elevation, and rest; ecchymosis usually does not require treatment unless severe.

■ Inflammation is the body's reaction to invasion by infectious agents or physical, chemical, or traumatic damage.

OUTLINE

I. The Skeletal System

   A. Bones of the skeleton are divided into two main parts: the axial skeleton, which includes the skull, spine, ribs, and sternum, and the appendicular skeleton, which includes the two limb girdles along with the attached limbs.

   B. Male bones tend to be larger and heavier than the female skeleton, and the female pelvic cavity is wider to accommodate childbirth.

   C. The skeleton plays a part in movement, support, and protection of internal organs; in blood cell production; and in storing for minerals, such as calcium and phosphorous.

II. Bones

   A. Bones consist of microscopic cells called osteocytes. Bone is made up of 35% organic material, 65% inorganic mineral salts, and water.

   B. The organic part derives from a protein called bone collagen.

   C. Bone formation

      1. The embryonic skeleton initially consists of collagenous protein fibers secreted by the osteoblasts.

      2. During the embryonic development, ossification begins. That is, mineral matter starts to replace previously formed cartilage, creating bone.

   D. Structure of the long bone contains a shaft, or diaphysis.

      1. At each end (extreme) of the diaphysis is an epiphysis.

      2. In the center of the shaft is the broad medullary canal or cavity, filled with yellow bone marrow, mostly made of fat cells.

      3. The medullary canal is surrounded by compact or hard bone that carries blood vessels to nourish the osteocytes.

      4. Where less strength is needed in the bone, some of the hard bone is dissolved away, leaving spongy bone.

      5. The outside of the bone is covered with the periosteum, which is necessary for bone growth, repair, and nutrition.

   E. Growth

      1. Osteoblasts are bone cells that deposit the new bone.

2. Osteoclasts are immense bone cells that secrete enzymes that digest the bony material, splitting off the bone minerals calcium and phosphorus, and enabling them to be absorbed by the surrounding fluid.

3. The length of a bone shaft continues to grow until all the epiphyseal plate cartilage is ossified.

F. Bone types

1. Bones are classified as one of four types on the basis of their shape: long bones, flat bones, irregular bones and short bones.

2. The degree of movement at a joint is determined by bone shape and joint structure.

III. Injuries to Bones

A. Fractures

1. A simple or closed fracture can be either incomplete or complete, but the broken ends of the bone do not penetrate the skin.

2. A compound or open fracture results in the fractured end penetrating the skin, greatly increasing the chances of wound and bone infection.

3. A greenstick fracture is an incomplete break, and is more common among children whose bones are more pliable than adults.

4. A comminuted fracture occurs when forces are great enough to shatter the bone into at least three pieces.

5. A stress fracture is a small, incomplete break due to overuse, poor muscle balance, lack of flexibility, weakness in soft tissues, or biomechanical problems. Lower leg and foot bones are particularly susceptible.

6. Epiphyseal plate fractures are breaks that occur near the epiphyseal (growth plate), especially in the wrist and ankle, mostly in individuals between 10 and 16 years of age due to sports participation.

7. Treatment involves the natural processes of bone remodeling, occurring with the broken bones held in their normal position relative to each other (reduction).

a. External fixation refers to the use of a cast to keep bones aligned.

b. Internal fixation occurs when surgery is necessary to keep bones aligned, often using wires, plates, and screws.

IV. Muscles

A. Muscle cells, like most cells of the body, are surrounded by a membrane called the sarcolemma, and are filled with a protein-rich cytoplasm called the sarcopolasm.

B. Skeletal muscles are very long and, unlike most of the body's cells, often have many nuclei. Skeletal muscle is attached to the bones of the body and is responsible for moving the bones relative to one another, under voluntary control.

C. Smooth muscle, which is not under conscious control and is not attached to the skeleton, is often found in the walls of hollow organs like the stomach, intestines, bladder, blood vessels, and uterus.

D. Cardiac muscle is found only in the heart, is not under conscious control, and even has the ability to contract without nerve stimulation.

E. Sphincter, or dilator, muscles are special circular muscles that open and close to control the passage of substances in various parts of the body.

V. Characteristics of Muscles

    A. Muscles are characterized by contractibility, the ability to shorten, unlike other body tissues.

    B Like nerve cells, muscle cells are excitable (irritable), meaning they are able to respond to electrical signals called action potentials (impulses).

    C. Muscles also exhibit characteristics of extensibility (the ability to be stretched) and elasticity (the ability to return to their original length after being stretched).

VI. Muscle Attachments and Functions

    A. Skeletal muscles are attached to a bone that does not move (origin) and a bone that does move (insertion). When the muscle contracts, since its volume cannot change, its belly gets thicker.

    B. Muscles are usually arranged in pairs, with the prime mover causing the main motion, and the antagonist opposing the main motion. Often other muscles, called synergists, are present to steady the movement of the larger muscles or to stabilize joint activity.

VII. Sources of Heat and Energy

VIII. Contraction of Skeletal Muscle

    A. Contraction of skeletal muscles within a motor unit occurs when the motor neuron, after receiving a nerve impulse from the central nervous system, releases a chemical neurotransmitter, acetylcholine, which diffuses across a gap known as the synaptic cleft (neuromuscular junction), to the muscle cell, which is stimulated to contract.

IX. Muscle Fatigue

    A. Muscle fatigue is caused by an accumulation of lactic acid in the muscles.

    B. If the muscle, which is always under a state of partial contraction (muscle tone), contracts too often, it will use up its oxygen reserves and start producing lactic acid, which causes muscle fatigue, or the reduction in a muscle's ability to contract and the generation of muscle pain.

X. Muscle Tone

    A. Muscle atrophy is the wasting away or loss of muscle tissue resulting from disease or lack of use. Vigorous exercise will reverse this type of problem unless it has gone too far. For athletes, immobilization because of injury is a common reason for lack of use.

    B. Muscle hypertrophy, which is an increase in the mass (size) of a muscle (the number of muscle fibers do not increase, but the fibers already present do increase in size), is commonly caused by exercise. For muscles to be enlarged beyond their normal size, they must be exposed to a training stimulus that is sufficient to cause overcompensation in the muscle.

XI. Injuries to Muscles

    A. A strain is caused by twisting or pulling a muscle or tendon.

        1. An acute strain is caused by trauma or an injury, improperly lifting heavy objects, or overstressing muscles.

        2. Chronic strains are usually the result of overuse—prolonged, repetitive movement of the muscles and tendons.

        3. Symptoms include pain, muscle spasm, muscle weakness, perhaps localized swelling, cramping or inflammation, and some loss of muscle function.

4. Treatment involves a first stage of reducing swelling and pain with rest, ice, compression, and elevation (RICE), a hard cast for moderate or severe injury, and perhaps surgery for some severe cases.

5. Rehabilitation, the second stage, involves an exercise program designed to prevent stiffness, improve range of motion, and restore the joint's normal flexibility and strength.

6. Lowering the risk of strains involves maintaining a healthy, well-balanced diet and a healthy weight, practicing safety measures to help prevent falls, wearing properly fitting shoes, replacing worn athletic shoes, doing stretching exercises daily, being in proper physical condition to play a sport, warming up and stretching before any sports or exercise, avoiding exercise or sports when tired or in pain, and running on even surfaces.

B. Sprains can result from a fall, a sudden twist, or a blow to the body that forces a joint out of its normal position, resulting in an overstretched ligament.

1. Typically sprains occur when people fall and land on an outstretched arm, slide into base, land on the side of their foot, or twist a knee with the foot planted firmly on the ground.

2. Usual symptoms include pain, swelling, bruising, and loss of the ability to move or use the joint.

3. Physicians grade sprains, with grade I being a mild sprain caused by overstretching or slight tearing of the ligaments with no joint instability. Grade II is a sprain with partial tearing of the ligament and is characterized by bruising, moderate pain, and swelling. Grade III is a severe tear or rupture of a ligament and accompanying severe pain, swelling, and bruising.

4. Rehabilitation and prevention are similar to that of a strain.

C. Tendonitis is an inflammation that occurs when tendons become irritated, most commonly from overuse.

1. Treatment includes avoiding the aggravating movements, and possibly some anti-inflammatory medications, icing, ultrasound therapy, and physical therapy.

2. To prevent the return of tendonitis, slowly increase the intensity and type of exercise, not trying to do more than the individual is ready for.

D. Bursitis is inflammation of the bursa (fluid-filled sacs that help reduce friction when joints move) often resulting from repetitive movement or prolonged or excessive pressure.

1. Treatment includes avoiding the activity that caused it, applying anti-inflammatory medications, or if necessary, drainage of the bursa, injection of cortisone and/or surgical excision.

2. To prevent bursitis from returning, strengthen muscles around the joint, avoid repetitive stress, cushion the joints, and take rest breaks.

E. A contusion is a direct blow or blunt injury that does not penetrate the skin, usually with a bruise from injury to blood vessels.

1. Mild contusions respond well to RICE (rest, ice, compression, elevation). Symptoms include swelling, pain when touched, redness, and ecchymosis.

2. If RICE is ineffective, a physician may prescribe physical therapy.

3. If a contusion is not managed properly, myositis ossificans, which is a calcification that forms within the muscle, can occur, usually requiring surgery to repair.

XII. Nerves

    A. Nerve tissue consists of two major types of nerve cells: neuroglia and neurons. Three types of neurons are found in the nervous system.

        1. Afferent (sensory) neurons carry nerve signals toward the central nervous system (brain and spinal cord).

        2. Efferent (motor) neurons carry nerve impulses away from the central nervous system to muscles and glands.

        3. Interneurons (associative neurons) carry nerve impulses from sensory neurons to motor neurons and make up most of the central nervous system.

    B. Neurons have the property of membrane excitability, meaning that they can create a voltage between the inside and outside of the neuron by pumping electrically charged atoms (ions). This voltage, when stimulated cannot only change, but it can move along the length of the neuron's fibers to the end of the axon fiber, where a synapse occurs and a neurotransmitter chemical transfers the electrical signal to another nerve cell or a muscle cell.

XIII. Injury to Nerves

    A. Injury to a nerve can stop signals to and from the brain, causing muscles not to work and loss of feeling in the injured area. This may be because the nerve is cut, experiencing pressure, or overstretched.

        1. If the insulating myelin sheath is sewn together where cut, the fibers may grow back out and restore function.

        2. If the insulation around the nerve was not cut, new fibers may grow down the empty insulator until reaching a muscle or sensory receptor.

        3. If both the nerve and insulation have been cut and the nerve not fixed, the new nerve fibers may grow into a ball at the end of the cut, forming a neuroma, which can be painful.

XIV. Soft Tissue Injuries

    A. Abrasions and scrapes occur when several layers of skin are torn loose or totally removed, exposing millions of nerve endings.

        1. Treatment includes washing with soap and water, removing all dirt and debris. If material is imbedded in the wound, it must be scraped. Pain medications may be necessary before cleaning. Antibiotic ointment is applied, and the wound is left open, unless oozing of fluid or blood is present.

            a. Loose skin flaps may be left in place if clean; if not, it should be removed carefully. Ice packs or cool towels can help relieve pain.

            b. The last tetanus immunization date should be checked. These should be given every 10 years.

        2. Seek medical attention if pain increases after several days, redness or red streaks appear beyond the edges, swelling occurs, or if there is purulent drainage (yellow, green, or bloody, foul-smelling pus).

    B. A laceration or cut is a tear in the skin that results from an injury. Most small lacerations (less than 1/4″ deep and 1/2″ long) can be treated at home without stitches.

        1. Lacerations need to be cleaned out with soap and water and irrigated well with clean water to remove any debris.

        a. To stop bleeding, cover the wound with a sterile gauze and apply direct and constant pressure. Immediate professional medical attention will be necessary if the bleeding is uncontrolled or spurts with a pulse.

        b. Bruising and swelling around the injury site may occur, for which ice can be applied with the area elevated above the heart.

    2. A physician should be contacted if the cut is deeper than 1/4″ and longer than 1/2″; the wound is in an area of the body that easily opens when moved; the wound is on the face, eyelids, or lips; if there are deep cuts on the palm, finger, elbow, or knee, and if there is any loss of sensation or normal range of motion as a result of the cut.

C. An avulsion is an injury in which layers of the skin are either torn off completely or a flap of skin remains, often accompanied by a great deal of bleeding. After cleaning, replace the flap of skin if it still is attached. If the skin is torn off completely, place it in a bag and on ice (keep it from getting frozen or soaked in water).

D. Puncture wounds are caused by sharp, pointed objects that penetrate the skin.

    1. To treat a puncture wound, first find out whether or not part of the object that caused the puncture is still in the wound, then determine whether other tissues (such as blood vessels, nerves, tendons, ligaments, bones, or internal organs) have been injured, then take steps to prevent infections.

    2. The risk of infection is greater if the penetrating object was exposed to soil, penetrated the sole of a shoe, or was injected into the skin under high pressure. If signs of infection occur, seek medical attention.

E. A hematoma is the formation of blood and tissue fluid that pools within a tissue space, a compartment, or an organ at any depth, and are usually the result of a contusion. Treatment is typically local compression and padding.

XV. The Body's Response to Injury

A. Inflammation is the body's initial response to invasion by an infectious agent or physical, chemical, or traumatic damage.

    1. An increase in blood supply is the result of blood vessel dilation.

    2. Increased capillary permeability permits molecules and cells larger than usual to escape from the capillaries.

    3. Leukocytes (white blood cells), including neutrophils, monocytes, and lymphocytes migrate from the capillaries to surrounding tissues. They release chemical mediators that control the accumulation and activation of other cells.

    4. Sometimes acute processes give way to a predominance of mononuclear phagocytes, a type of white blood cell good at mopping up.

B. Cell regeneration allows wounds to heal, as they divide and replace the damaged cells. If the damage is severe enough, damaged tissue is replaced by fibrous or scar tissue.

C. Cellular dedifferentiation is the term used to describe mature, differentiated cells that reenter the cell cycle so they can proliferate to produce more cells of the same function.

D. Cellular transdifferentiation describes a regeneration process where cells can dedifferentiate, divide, then differentiate into cells of a different type and function. This is particularly useful in damaged organs that have lost some of their function.

E. Tissue remodeling describes the process in which cells and molecules are modified and reassembled, building a new composition of cell types and extracellular matrix (ECM).

1. First, new blood vessels form (angiogenesis), spanning the wound.
2. Fibroblasts migrate and proliferate, filling and bridging the wound.
3. The ECM is deposited.

F. During the remodeling stage, collagen fibers are thickened and strengthened and lost cells and tissue are replaced by connective tissue.

VOCABULARY REVIEW

Matching

Match the terms on the right with the definitions on the left. Terms may be used once, more than once, or not at all.

_____ 1. The space between adjacent neurons, or a neuron and muscle fiber, through which an impulse is transmitted by chemical messenger

_____ 2. A break in the bone at the growth plate; typically at the wrist or ankle

_____ 3. The end of a long bone

_____ 4. The central part of a muscle

_____ 5. A muscle that helps steady a joint

_____ 6. Inflammation of the tendon

_____ 7. Bones of the pelvic and shoulder girdles as well as the limbs

_____ 8. The bones of the head and trunk (skull, spine, sternum, and ribs)

_____ 9. The type of muscle that makes up the heart

_____ 10. A protein substance found in bone and cartilage

_____ 11. A break in the bone in which the bone ends are shattered in many pieces

_____ 12. The chemical released when a nerve impulse is transmitted to the muscle

_____ 13. The electric change occurring across the membrane of a nerve or muscle cell during transmission of a nerve impulse

_____ 14. A muscle whose action opposes the action of another muscle

A. acetylcholine
B. action potential
C. angiogenesis
D. antagonist
E. appendicular skeleton
F. avulsion
G. axial skeleton
H. belly
I. bursitis
J. cardiac muscle
K. collagen fibers
L. comminuted fracture
M. compound fracture
N. connective tissue
O. contractibility
P. contusion
Q. diaphysis
R. ecchymosis
S. elasticity
T. epiphyseal plate fracture
U. epiphysis
V. excitability
W. extensibility
X. external fixation
Y. extracellular matrix (ECM)

_____ 15. A complete break in the bone in which the bone ends separate and break through the skin; also known as an open fracture

_____ 16. Cells whose secretions support and connect organs and tissues in the body

_____ 17. The ability to shorten or reduce the distance between the parts

_____ 18. The shaft of a long bone

_____ 19. The ability to return to original form after being compressed or stretched

_____ 20. Inflammation of the bursa

_____ 21. The ability to respond to stimuli; also known as irritability

_____ 22. An incomplete break in the shaft of the bone usually occurring in children

_____ 23. The part of the skeletal muscle that is attached to the movable part of a bone

_____ 24. Surgical alignment of bones to maintain alignment for the purpose of reduction

_____ 25. The ability to respond to stimuli; also known as excitability

_____ 26. The muscle cell membrane

_____ 27. The material within the muscle cell, excluding the nucleus

_____ 28. A break in the bone that may be complete or incomplete but does not break through the skin; also known as a closed fracture

_____ 29. The type of muscle attached to a bone, or bones, of the skeleton and aids in body movements; also known as voluntary or striated muscle

_____ 30. The type of muscle that is not attached to bone and is nonstriated and involuntary; also known as visceral

_____ 31. A type of circular muscle

_____ 32. The center of the shaft of a long bone

_____ 33. A motor nerve plus all of the muscle fibers it stimulates

_____ 34. The result of accumulation of lactic acid in the muscle

Z. greenstick fracture

AA. hematoma

BB. inflammation

CC. insertion

DD. internal fixation

EE. irritability

FF. medullary canal

GG. membrane excitability

HH. motor unit

II. muscle fatigue

JJ. muscle tone

KK. myelin sheath

LL. myositis ossificans

MM. neuromuscular junction

NN. origin

OO. ossification

PP. osteoblasts

QQ. osteoclasts

RR. osteocyte

SS. periosteum

TT. prime mover

UU. reduction

VV. regeneration

WW. remodeling

XX. sarcolemma

YY. sarcoplasm

ZZ. scar tissue

AAA. simple fracture

BBB. skeletal muscle

CCC. smooth muscle

DDD. sphincter muscle

EEE. spongy bone

FFF. sprain

GGG. strain

HHH. stress fracture

III. synapse

JJJ. synergist

KKK. tendonitis

_____ 35. The state of partial contraction in which muscles are maintained.

_____ 36. A calcification that forms within the muscle, resulting from an improperly managed contusion

_____ 37. The part of the skeletal muscle that is attached to the fixed part of a bone

_____ 38. The ability to lengthen and increase the distance between two parts

_____ 39. The use of a cast to maintain proper alignment of bones for the purpose of reduction

_____ 40. Noncellular material that separates connective tissue cells

_____ 41. The type of bone cell involved in the resorption of bony tissue

_____ 42. A bone cell

_____ 43. The fibrous tissue that covers the bone

_____ 44. The muscle that provides movement in a single direction

_____ 45. The process of putting broken bones back into their proper alignment

_____ 46. The process of absorbing and replacing bone in the skeletal system.

_____ 47. A lattice-like arrangement of bony plates found largely near the ends of long bones

_____ 48. An injury resulting from a fall, sudden twist, or blow to the body that forces a joint out of its normal position

_____ 49. The process of bone formation

_____ 50. The type of bone cell involved in the formation of bony tissue

Crossword Puzzle

Identify the terms described in the puzzle clues, then write the letters in the boxes. (Many terms are more than one word.)

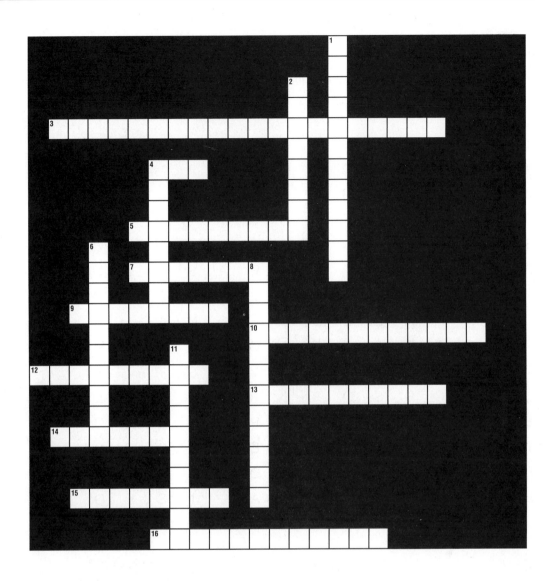

Across
3. when cells create new cells with a different function _____
4. substance secreted by connective tissue (abbr.) _____
5. white blood cell _____
7. growth of nerve fibers into a ball _____
9. blood and tissue fluid pools within a tissue _____
10. pain, heat, redness, and swelling _____
12. injury from a direct blow not interrupting the skin _____
13. bruising _____
14. the space between adjacent neurons _____

15. several skin layers are torn loose _____
16. act of wound healing _____

Down
1. a nerve fiber insulator _____
2. a sharp object penetrates the skin _____
4. a neuron carrying messages away from the brain or spinal cord _____
6. also known as a cut _____
8. formation of new blood cells _____
11. a type of tissue whose secretions support and connect organs _____

Word Search Puzzle

Several human muscle names from this chapter can be found among the letters of the word search puzzle. How many can you find? (Many terms are more than one word.)

```
C  S  B  R  V  S  S  U  E  T  U  L  G  W  E
W  B  T  R  A  P  E  Z  I  U  S  A  M  U  T
B  H  A  M  S  T  R  I  N  G  S  T  Q  B  R
D  F  M  B  T  R  X  Q  C  S  I  I  V  N  I
S  S  Q  A  U  T  C  F  U  D  L  S  Q  R  C
E  I  I  H  S  Y  P  I  Z  B  A  S  F  Z  E
R  B  L  L  S  R  E  O  L  R  I  D  S  P
R  I  K  A  A  O  E  L  T  E  O  M  I  I  S
A  C  U  T  T  R  A  T  A  O  T  U  O  L  U
T  E  A  R  E  N  O  U  E  V  C  S  T  I  E
U  P  A  C  R  S  O  P  I  R  E  D  L  C  L
S  S  T  E  A  X  O  R  M  P  P  O  E  A  O
T  U  T  V  L  N  O  G  F  E  L  R  D  R  S
S  X  S  U  I  M  E  N  C  O  T  S  A  G  S
E  F  B  V  S  T  I  B  I  A  L  I  S  L  O
```

BICEPS	DELTOID	GLUTEUS
FRONTALIS	HAMSTRINGS	LATISSIMUSDORSI
GRACILIS	PECTORALIS	RECTUS
MASSETER	SERRATUS	SOLEUS
SARTORIUS	TIBIALIS	TRAPEZIUS
TEMPORALIS	VASTUSLATERALIS	
TRICEPS	EXTERNALOBLIQUE	

ANATOMY IDENTIFICATION

1. Color and label each different bone or groups of bones (examples of groups would be the ribs, metacarpals, phalanges, etc). Each bone or group of bones should be colored with the same color (for example, there is a right humerus and a left humerus, but both humerus bones should be colored the same color).

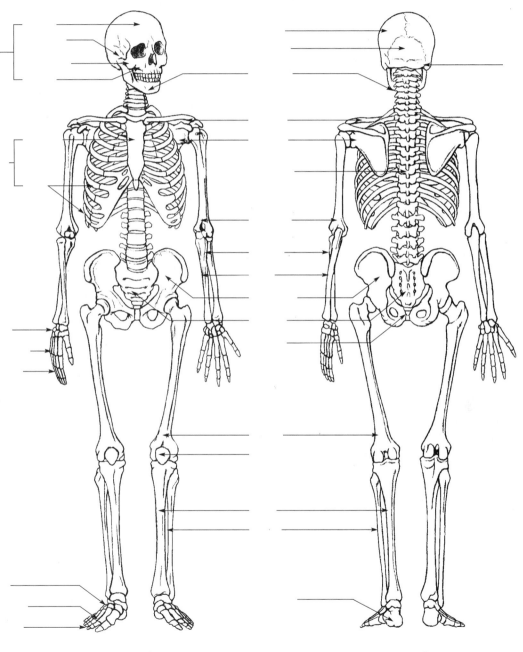

A. Anterior   **B. Posterior**

2. Label all anatomical parts on the diagram. Color the articular cartilage, spongy bone, yellow marrow, and periosteum.

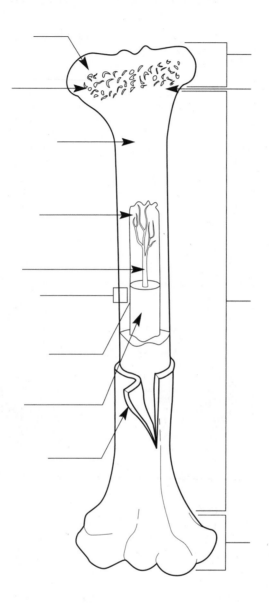

3. Color all muscles on the next two pages in such a way that muscles with the same name are colored with the same color (for example, the right pectoralis major would be the same color as the left pectoralis major). The same color can be used for different muscles if you run short on different colors, as long as the different muscles are not bordering each other.

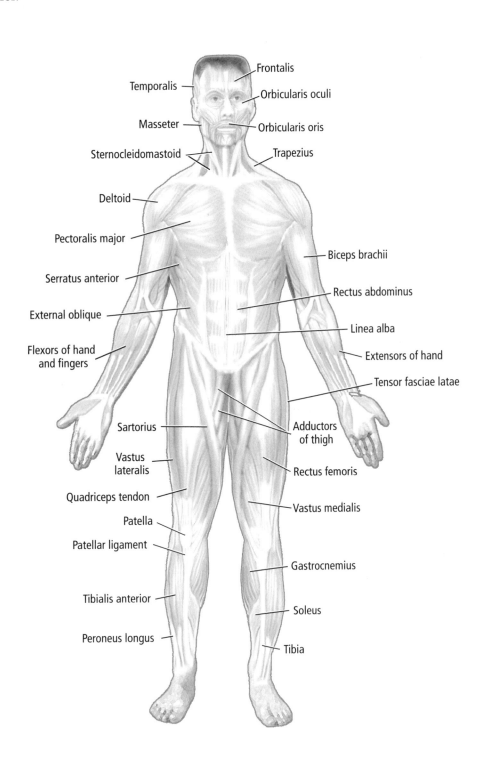

Frontalis
Temporalis
Orbicularis oculi
Masseter
Orbicularis oris
Sternocleidomastoid
Trapezius
Deltoid
Pectoralis major
Biceps brachii
Serratus anterior
Rectus abdominus
External oblique
Linea alba
Flexors of hand and fingers
Extensors of hand
Tensor fasciae latae
Sartorius
Adductors of thigh
Vastus lateralis
Rectus femoris
Quadriceps tendon
Vastus medialis
Patella
Patellar ligament
Gastrocnemius
Tibialis anterior
Soleus
Peroneus longus
Tibia

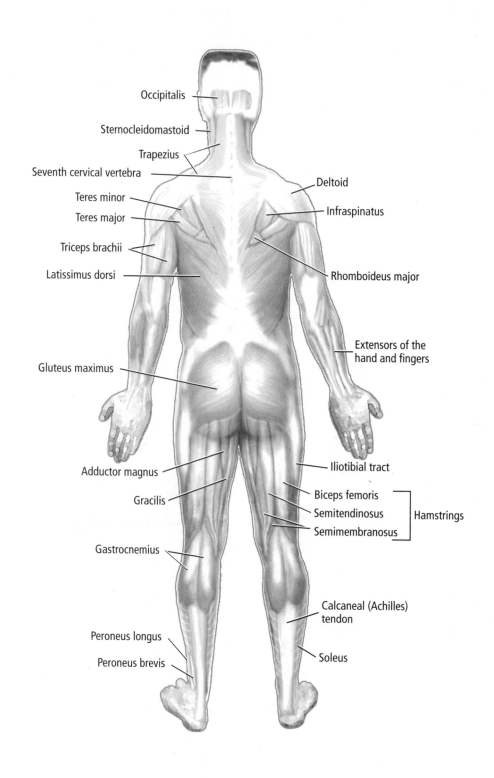

Occipitalis

Sternocleidomastoid

Trapezius

Seventh cervical vertebra

Teres minor

Teres major

Triceps brachii

Latissimus dorsi

Deltoid

Infraspinatus

Rhomboideus major

Extensors of the hand and fingers

Gluteus maximus

Adductor magnus

Gracilis

Gastrocnemius

Peroneus longus

Peroneus brevis

Iliotibial tract

Biceps femoris

Semitendinosus

Semimembranosus

Hamstrings

Calcaneal (Achilles) tendon

Soleus

ACTIVITIES

1. Look closely at a full-sized skeleton. Learn the names of all skeletal parts identified on diagrams in the workbook.

   _____

   _____

   _____

   _____

2. Study photographs of different kinds of soft tissue injuries to the point where you can recognize the type of injury or at least narrow down the possibilities when such wounds are encountered in the field. Be ready to describe the treatment you would provide in each case.

   _____

   _____

   _____

   _____

   _____

ONLINE RESEARCH

■ Research different products that are commercially available for the treatment of soft tissue injuries. Discuss similarities and differences of the products? If possible, investigate the price of each product, and write an analysis of which products give you the desired results for the least cost.

   _____

   _____

   _____

   _____

   _____

CHAPTER 17

The Foot, Ankle, and Lower Leg

KEY CONCEPTS

■ The foot has three arches: transverse, a medial longitudinal, and a lateral longitudinal; the foot has 26 bones (7 tarsals, 5 metatarsals, and 14 phalanges); the foot has 38 joints; the ankle joint is made up of the talocrural and subtalar joints; there are five main ligaments in the ankle, anterior talofibular, anterior tibiofibular, calcaneofibular, posterior talofibular, and the deltoid.

■ The intrinsic muscles cause movement of the toes and help support the arches of the foot. The extrinsic muscles aid in the movement of the ankle and foot. Table 17-1 lists the names and functions of each muscle of the lower leg and foot.

Table 17-1 Muscles Moving the Foot and Toes

Muscles Moving the Foot

MUSCLE	FUNCTION
Gastrocnemius	Plantar flexes foot, flexes leg, supinates foot
Soleus	Plantar flexes foot
Tibialis posterior	Plantar flexes foot
Tibialis anterior	Dorsally flexes foot
Peroneus tertius	Dorsally flexes foot
Peroneus longus	Everts, plantar flexes foot
Peroneus brevus	Everts foot
Plantaris	Plantar flexes foot

Muscles Moving the Toes

MUSCLE	FUNCTION
Flexor hallucis brevis	Flexes great toe
Flexor hallucis longus	Flexes great toe
Extensor hallucis longus	Extends great toe, dorsiflexes ankle
Interossei dorsales	Abduct, flex toes
Flexor digitorum longus	Flexes toes, extends foot
Extensor digitorum longus	Extends toes
Abductor hallucis	Abducts, flexes great toe
Abductor digiti minimi	Abducts little toe

(continues)

(continued)

- ■ Common injuries:
  - Ankle sprains are usually the result of excessive inversion or plantar flexion. Sprains are treated with cold, compression, and elevation.
  - Arch sprains result from overstretched ligaments in the arch, which then cannot support the foot and absorb shocks. Sprains are treated with cold, compression, and elevation.
  - Blisters result from friction that causes the layers of the skin to separate; fluid seeps in between the layer and creates the blister. Blisters should be covered and padded.
  - Turf toe is caused by hyperextension of the great toe. It is treated with ice, rest, compression, elevation, and support.
  - Plantar faciitis is a strain on the ligamentous tissues in the bottom of the foot due to chronic overuse, overstretching, and irritation. Treatment is targeted at correcting training errors, ice, and massage.
  - Heel bruises occur due to repeated stress. They are treated with cold application, elevation, and padding.
  - Heel spurs are bony growths on the calcaneus that cause painful inflammation of the soft tissues. Management includes taping the arch and using shoe inserts.
  - Fractures are breaks in the bones. Treatment must be sought from a physician and will depend on the severity of the break.
  - Contusions are injuries to the soft tissues.
  - The exact causes of muscle cramps is unknown. Cramps can be relieved by passive stretching, fluid replacement, massage, rest, and ice.
  - Achilles tendonitis is an inflammation of the Achilles tendon. The best treatment is prevention by stretching before beginning exercise.
  - An Achilles tendon rupture is a complete tear of the tendon. This injury usually requires surgical treatment.
- ■ Medial tibial stress syndrome, or shin splints, is pain that occurs in the lower portion of the leg. Treatment consists of icing, reducing activity levels, and gentle stretching,
  - Stress fractures are microscopic breaks in the bone due to repeated stress and overuse. Treatment from a physician should be sought.
  - Compartment syndrome is damage to tissues resulting from swelling of one or more of the compartments in the legs. Immediate emergency treatment should be sought.

OUTLINE

I. The Lower Leg

  A. Even with protection, the lower leg will still be susceptible to injury.

  B. Common injuries include contusions, strains, tendonitis, tendon ruptures, medial tibial stress syndrome (shin splints), stress fractures, compartment syndrome, and fractures.

II. The Foot and Ankle
   A. About 15% of all sports injuries involve the ligaments, bones, and tendons of the ankle.
   B. Feet can suffer from rather minor conditions that are often just as debilitating as the more serious foot problems, such as athlete's foot, turf toe, calluses, ingrown toenails, and blisters.
   C. Basic Anatomy of the Foot and Ankle
      1. The key to the foot's function is a set of three arches, which help in absorbing the impact of walking, running, and jumping.
         a. The medial longitudinal arch is the highest and most important; composed of the calcaneus, talus, navicular, cuneiforms, and the first three metatarsals.
         b. The lateral longitudinal arch is lower and flatter and composed of the calcaneus, talus, cuboid, and fourth and fifth metatarsals,
         c. The transverse arch is composed of the cuneiforms, the cuboid, and the five metatarsal bases.
      2. The foot consists of 7 tarsals, 5 metatarsals, and 14 phalanges. The tarsal bones consist of the talus, calcaneus, navicular, cuboid, and the medial, intermediate, and lateral cuneiform bones.
      3. The ankle joint is formed by a combination of two joints.
         a. The talocrural joint is made up of the tibia, fibula, and talus. It is a hinge joint making dorsiflexion and plantar flexion possible.
         b. The subtalar joint is made up of the talus and calcaneus. It can move around the oblique axis.
         c. Large bony prominences, called malleoli, are located on either side of the ankle.
      4. Ligaments of the foot and ankle most commonly injured are the anterior talofibular, anterior tibiofibular, calcaneofibular, posterior talofibular, and deltoid.
III. Basic Anatomy of the Lower Leg
   A. Muscles of the lower leg and foot have two classifications.
      1. Intrinsic muscles are located within the foot and cause movement of the toes (plantar flexors, dorsiflexors, abductors, adductors of the toes). Several also help support the arches.
      2. Extrinsic muscles are located outside the foot and have long tendons that cross the ankle and attach to the bones of the foot, except for the talus which has no tendon attachments.
IV. Common Injuries of the Foot and Ankle
   A. Ankle sprains are one of the most common injuries among the population and are very common among athletes, mostly due to a combination of excessive inversion and plantar flexion.
      1. The most commonly injured ligament is the anterior talofibular ligament.
      2. Less common is the eversion sprain because of the protective function of the deltoid ligament.

B. Both inversion and eversion sprains are categorized into three groups.

1. In a *first-degree (mild) sprain*, one or more of the supporting ligaments are stretched, with minor discomfort, point tenderness, little or no swelling, and no abnormal movement in the joint.

2. In a *second-degree (moderate) sprain*, a portion of one or more ligaments is torn, with pain, swelling, point tenderness, disability, loss of function, and slight abnormal movement.

3. In a *third-degree (severe) sprain*, one or more ligaments have been completely torn, with extreme pain (unless there is nerve damage when there may be little pain), loss of function, point tenderness, rapid swelling, and the chance of an accompanying fracture.

C. Arch sprains, most of which involve the metatarsal or inner longitudinal arch, reduce the ability of the arches to absorb shock as well as they should.

1. Arch sprains are caused by overuse, overweight, fatigue, training on hard surfaces, and wearing nonsupportive, worn shoes.

2. Treatment of arch sprains includes cold, compression, and elevation.

D. Blisters in athletes often occur on the feet as layers of skin rub together and friction causes separation. Fluid then forms in the separation, creating pressure on nerve endings.

1. A broken blister creates an open wound and is susceptible to infection.

2. If the blister is small and intact, treatment is usually not necessary. Otherwise the blister should be covered with a bandage and changed daily.

3. Prevention of blisters involves eliminating friction by selecting the appropriate shoe and sock and the right size and type for the sport.

E. Great toe sprain (turf toe) often involves the foot sliding backward on a slippery surface, which forcefully hyperextends the big toe.

1. Immediate care includes protection, rest, ice, compression, elevation, and support.

2. The physician may x-ray to rule out more severe injury, but most sprains of the big toe are minor.

F. Plantar fasciitis usually involves overuse of the plantar fascia, and may be caused by unsupportive footwear, a tight Achilles tendon, or running on hard surfaces.

1. The athlete with plantar fasciitis will experience pain and tenderness on the bottom of the foot near the heel.

2. Treatment involves correcting training errors, changing shoes, icing, and massage.

G. Heel bruise is one of the more disabling contusions in athletics. The heel must be protected during physical activity.

1. Cold application before the activity, and cold and elevation afterward, can help reduce swelling and pain.

2. Heel cups can help protect against the heel's impact with the ground or floor.

H. The heel spur is a bony growth on the calcaneus that causes painful inflammation of the accompanying soft tissue and is treated by taping the arch or using shoe inserts to help reduce the pull of the plantar fascia.

I. Fractures of the foot and ankle immediately impair the athlete's performance in most sporting activities. Often a site of point tenderness is present and an obvious deformity seen. It is important to complete a thorough examination of the involved extremity to avoid incorrect assessment.

V. Rehabilitation of Foot and Ankle Injuries

    A. The best way to determine when healing is complete is by the absence of pain.

    B. Before the beginning of any rehabilitation exercise program, the certified athletic trainer should consult with the sports medicine team to establish an individual program tailored for that individual athlete and the specific sports injury to be rehabilitated.

VI. Common Injuries of the Lower Leg

    A. Contusions occur most often over the shin, where the tibia is just below the skin and sensitive to direct trauma. The muscular areas of the leg may also suffer from contusions.

        1. A possible complication is significant swelling within the various compartments, which may lead to compartment syndrome.

        2. Damage to the peroneal nerve may also occur, with transient tingling and numbness to the lateral surface of the leg or dorsal surface of the foot. Symptoms are often temporary and recovery is usually complete.

    B. Strains are usually the result of violent contraction, overstretching, or continued overuse, most commonly involving the calf muscles near the musculotendinous junction or at the insertion of the Achilles tendon.

    C. A muscle cramp is a sudden, involuntary contraction of a muscle. Although the cause is unknown, several factors may contribute to their incidence.

        1. Fatigue by working the muscle beyond it limits.

        2. After a fracture heals, an atrophied muscle is more likely to cramp if it is not strengthened to preinjury status.

        3. Lack of fluids, which can cause dehydration and lessen the ability of the body to cool itself.

        4. Electrolyte (mineral) imbalance of sodium, magnesium, calcium, or potassium.

        5. Poor flexibility

        6. Improperly fitted equipment that causes excessive strain.

        7. Treatment includes passive stretching, fluid replacement, massage, rest, and ice. Passive stretching will help keep the muscle from forcefully shortening.

    D. Achilles tendonitis usually involves tearing of the tissues of the Achilles tendon caused by excessive stress.

        1. Inflammation may be due to a single incident or from an accumulation of smaller stresses that produce numerous small tears over time.

        2. Symptoms usually develop gradually and discomfort is usually attributed to the aches and pains that normally accompany muscle fatigue. In severe cases, the tendon ruptures causing severe pain and making walking virtually impossible.

        3. Treatment involves preventing inflammation by stretching the Achilles tendon before exercise to help maintain flexibility. Chronic Achilles tendonitis should be assessed by a sports medicine physician or podiatrist.

        4. Other methods of treatment include icing, anti-inflammatory medications, physical therapy, and rest.

E. Achilles tendon ruptures must be surgically repaired, with rehabilitation taking up to a year before the athlete is ready to return to play.

F. Medial tibial stress syndrome (shin splints) is a catchall term for pain that occurs below the knee either on the front outside part of the leg (anterior shin splints) or on the inside of the leg (medial shin splints).

　1. Shin splints are normally the result of doing too much too soon, often occurring early in the training program.

　2. Medial shin splints include the tightness of the gastrocnemius and soleus muscles, placing additional strain on the tibialis anterior muscle. Worn or ill-fitting shoes increase the stress on the leg muscles, whereas softer surfaces and shoe cushioning materials absorb more shock.

　3. Treatment includes icing immediately after practice or competition, reducing the activity level, and gentle stretching of the posterior leg muscles. Physical therapy, orthotics devices, anti-inflammatory medications, and a strengthening and flexibility program help correct muscle imbalance.

G. A stress fracture is an incomplete crack in the bone, which is a far more serious injury than shin splints, but may have many of the same symptoms.

　1. Stress fractures are microscopic, but may lead to a full fracture if left untreated.

　2. A "hot spot" of sharp, intense pain along the shin when touched is a good sign of a possible stress fracture. Usually stress fractures feel better the next morning, but shin splints feel worse.

H. Compartment syndrome results from a swelling in one of the four lower leg compartments. The four compartments are the anterior compartment, peroneal compartment, deep posterior compartment, and superficial posterior compartment.

　1. Causes of the swelling could be contusions, fractures, crushing injuries, localized infection, excessive exercise, or overstretching.

　2. Initial symptoms are point tenderness and pain of the muscle group involved, then in later stages numbness, weakness, and the inability to use the muscle. Compartment syndrome must be diagnosed immediately because of the possible neurological, muscular, or vascular damage that may occur and may be irreversible.

　3. For treatment, the injured person must be immediately transported to the nearest medical facility.

I. Fractures of the tibia are usually readily recognized because it is the weight-bearing bone of the lower leg. Fractures of the fibula present tenderness, local swelling, increased pain, but might be mistaken for a contusion, since walking is still possible.

VII. Additional Tests for the Foot, Ankle, and Lower Leg

A. The anterior drawer test determines the integrity of the anterior talofibular ligament.

B. The plantar fascia test locates plantar fascia pain.

C. The talar tilt test determines the integrity of the calcaneofibular ligament.

D. Tinel's sign method tests the tibial nerve.

VOCABULARY REVIEW

Matching

Match the terms on the right with the definitions on the left. Terms may be used once, more than once, or not at all.

_____ 1. A ligament that connects the tibia to the fibula in front of the ankle

_____ 2. A condition that develops when swelling exists in one or more of the four compartments of the leg or arm

_____ 3. A joint in the ankle found between the tibia, fibula, and talus

_____ 4. One of the three arches of the foot, composed of the calcaneus, talus, navicular, cuneiforms, and the first three metatarsals

_____ 5. A sudden, involuntary contraction of a muscle

_____ 6. The lower leg deep posterior compartment; contains the popliteus, flexor digitorum longus, flexor hallucis longus, and tibialis posterior muscles

_____ 7. A tendon in the back of the ankle and foot that attaches the gastrocnemius and soleus muscles to the calcaneus.

_____ 8. A joint in the ankle found between the talus and calcaneus

_____ 9. The lower leg superficial posterior compartment; contains the gastrocnemius, soleus, and plantaris muscles

_____ 10. Pain that occurs below the knee either on the front, outside portion of the leg or the inside of the leg; also known as shin splints

_____ 11. The lower leg peroneal compartment; contains the peroneus longus and peroneus brevis muscles

_____ 12. Referring to muscles that are outside a body part, organ, or bone

_____ 13. The highest arch of the foot

_____ 14. Referring to muscles that are inside a body part, organ, or bone

_____ 15. One of the three arches of the foot composed of the calcaneus, talus, cuboid, and the fourth and fifth metatarsals

A. Achilles tendon
B. anterior compartment
C. anterior tibiofibular ligament
D. calcaneofibular ligament
E. compartment syndrome
F. cramp
G. deep posterior compartment
H. deltoid ligament
I. extrinsic muscles
J. intrinsic muscles
K. lateral longitudinal arch
L. malleoli
M. medial longitudinal arch
N. medial tibial stress syndrome
O. peroneal compartment
P. plantar fascia
Q. posterior tibiofibular ligament
R. shin splints
S. subtalar joint
T. superficial posterior compartment
U. talocrural joint
V. transverse arch

_____ 16. Wide, nonelastic ligamentous tissue that extends from the anterior portion of the calcaneus to the heads of the metatarsals

_____ 17. The lower leg anterior compartment; contains the tibialis anterior, extensor digitorum longus, peroneus tertius, and extensor hallucis muscles

_____ 18. A commonly injured ligament that is triangular in shape and consists of a superficial and deep layer, which connect the talus to the medial malleolus

_____ 19. The large bony prominences located on either side of the ankle

_____ 20. A ligament that connects the tibia to the fibula on the back side of the ankle

_____ 21. Pain that occurs below the knee either on the front, outside portion of the leg or the inside of the leg; also known as medial tibial stress syndrome

_____ 22. One of the three arches of the foot composed of the cuneiforms, the cuboid, and the fifth metatarsal bones

ANATOMY IDENTIFICATION

1. Label and color the different bones of the foot. Color all the bones that have the same name the same color (for example, all distal phalanges should be one color and the middle phalanges another). Use brackets to show the three major bone groupings of the foot.

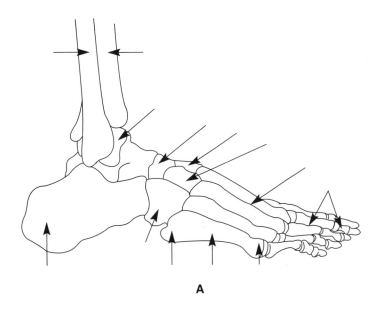

A

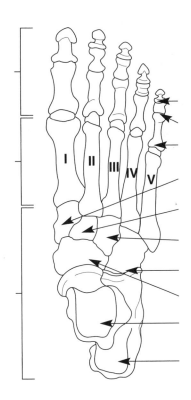

B

2. Label all structural parts of the foot and lower leg, front, side, and back views. Color the
different muscles with different colors. If the same muscle is pictured in different views,
use the same color for each. Also, use the same color for a muscle's tendon that you used
for the muscle.

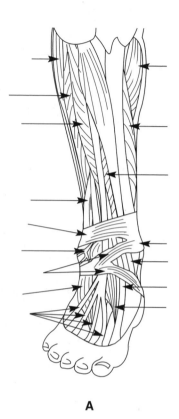

A

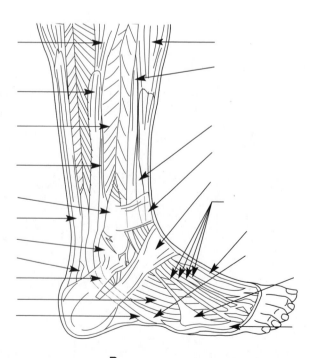

B

2. (continued)

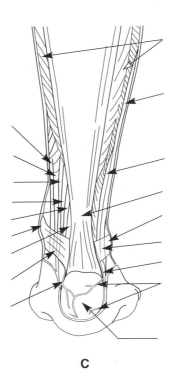

c

ACTIVITIES

1. Examine a model of an ankle and foot that shows ligament and/or tendon connections. Identify all structures referred to in the textbook. Then teach someone else the structure of the foot and ankle without looking at notes, diagrams, or any other outside sources.

_____

_____

_____

_____

_____

2. Demonstrate, by moving your own foot and ankle, the different actions of muscles and connecting tendons of the ankle and foot.

_____

_____

_____

_____

_____

ONLINE RESEARCH

■ Research current or alternative treatments of the ankle and foot that differ from those mentioned in the textbook. Identify which are improvements and which are just variations of the same procedure.

_____

_____

_____

_____

_____

■ Foot and lower leg structure is also very important to other mammals. Choose three other mammals and research what is different and what is the same about their foot structure and function.

_____

_____

_____

_____

_____

CHAPTER 18

The Knee

(continued)

- Meniscus tears, which are caused by sudden twisting of the knee. Immediate treatment should be application of ice and a compressive wrap.
- Epiphyseal injuries, which may result in alteration in the length of the bones involved.
- Osgood-Schlatter condition, a group of symptoms involving the tibial tubercle epiphysis. To prevent the problem from worsening, address the pain, swelling, and flexibility.
- Iliotibial band syndrome, an inflammation of the iliotibial band that usually occurs over the knee joint. Treatment for this syndrome involves assessing and correcting problems of gait and training.
- Fractures of the knee, which are the result of high-energy trauma.

OUTLINE

I. The Knee
  A. Because the knee supports the majority of the body weight, it is at risk of overuse in both contact and noncontact sports.
  B. The knee is composed of three major bones and muscle groups.
    1. The bone of the upper leg is the femur, distally formed into a pair of rounded prominences (condyles) and the lower leg provides the tibia and fibula. The proximal flat surface of the tibia is called the tibial plateau.
    2. The tibiofemoral joint is a weight-bearing, hinge joint, held together with a joint capsule and several ligaments.
  C. Cartilage, in the form of articular cartilage covers the ends of the tibia and femur, providing a smooth surface for gliding. Two crescent-shaped wedges, called menisci, are also found between the tibia and femur.
    1. The medial meniscus is between the medial femoral condyle and the medial tibial plateau.
    2. The lateral meniscus is between the lateral femoral condyle and the lateral tibial plateau.
    3. The two menisci aid in shock absorption, distributing forces, and improving stability.
    4. They are bathed in synovial fluid produced by the synovial membrane of the knee joint.
  D. Ligaments of the knee connect the tibia and femur together.
    1. The medial collateral ligament (MCL) is outside the joint capsule and attaches to the femur above and tibia below, providing medial stability.
    2. The lateral collateral ligament (LCL) is outside the joint capsule and attaches to the femur and the head of the fibula, providing lateral stability.
    3. The anterior cruciate ligament (ACL) is within the capsule and attaches to the femur and the anterior aspect of the tibial plateau, restricting translation (anterior movement) of the tibia on the femur.

4. The posterior cruciate ligament (PCL) is within the capsule and attaches to the femur and the posterior aspect of the tibial plateau, resisting posterior translation of the tibia on the femur.

5. The ACL and PCL cross over each other with the ACL running **A**nterior-to-**P**osterior-**Ex**ternally (APEX) and the PCL running **P**osterior-to-**A**nterior-**In**ternally (PAIN).

E. The patellofemoral joint includes the patella (kneecap), which rides in the trochlear groove on the distal end of the femur, and is a sesamoid (plate-shaped) bone enveloped within the quadriceps tendon.

1. The patella gives a mechanical advantage to extending the knee, increasing the quadriceps force by 33% to 50%.

2. The retropatellar (backside of the patella) surface is covered with a thick layer of articular cartilage.

3. The quadricep muscles, quadriceps tendon, patella, and patellar tendon comprise the structures of the extensor mechanism of the knee joint.

F. Muscles that move the leg are the strongest in the body.

1. The vastus medialis, vastus intermedius, vastus lateralis, and rectus femoris, collectively known as the quadriceps, extend the knee.

2. The sartorius and gracilis are strap-like muscles of the thigh that assist with flexion of the knee and are attached distally to the anteriomedial tibia near the semitendinosus distal attachment in an area know as the pes ansurine.

3. The hamstrings (medial: semitendinosus and semimembranosus; lateral: biceps femoris) attach to the pelvis and femur proximally and insert onto the posterior tibia, and flex the knee joint and extend the hip joint.

II. Knee Injuries

A. Patellofemoral problems are some of the most challenging for both athlete and trainer because it is not easy to identify as the source of the problem.

1. The classic complaint is aching pain in front of the knee. There may be a grinding noise (crepitus), with mild or no swelling. The patella may appear to face inward instead of forward. Patellofemoral provocation tests, such as a forward lunge or step-down test, can reproduce the pain the athlete is complaining of. Comparison to the uninvolved side is always recommended.

2. Treatment involves correcting the suspected cause, such as support with a shoe insert, or low-dye taping. Strengthening exercises that do not cause pain. Sometimes braces and specialized taping of the patella can make the patient more comfortable during rehabilitation.

B. Patellar tendonitis is often seen in sports that involve jumping. It is sometimes called jumper's knee.

1. Symptoms include anterior knee pain below the patella over the patellar tendon.

2. Activity modification should be considered to allow the tendon time to heal. Non-impact activities such as cycling and swimming will allow the patellar tendon to heal.

C. Fat pad syndrome involves a region of fatty tissue lying deep to the patellar tendon, also known as Hoffa's fat pad. It can become inflamed and may be confused with patellar tendonitis.

1. Activities that require rapidly kicking the knee into full extension should be avoided.

2. Specialized taping, icing, and anti-inflammatory medications may help.

D. Medial collateral ligament (MCL) strain often results from stretching and a valgus (outward) force to the medial tibiofemoral joint.

    1. Symptoms include pain and tenderness felt on the medial aspect of the knee, and difficulty bearing weight on the leg with acute grade II and III sprains, limited motion in full flexion and extension, swelling of the medial knee.

    2. Treatment of acute injuries is with PRICE (protection, rest, ice, compression, elevation), with the protection consisting of a protective wrap, brace, or crutches. Bending and extending the knee in pain-free ranges can occur until the knee obtains 110 to 115 degrees of flexion when cycling may be initiated.

E. Lateral collateral ligament sprain can occur with a blow to the medial side of the knee resulting in a varus (inside) stress to the knee joint.

    1. Tenderness is common with palpation. Pain and laxity will be present with a varus stress test.

    2. Treatment is similar to MCL sprains.

F. Torn anterior cruciate ligament (ACL) is a more common injury among females in sports like basketball and soccer than in males.

    1. Females tend to place more emphasis on the quadriceps muscles than male athletes.

    2. There is no hormonal factor involved in the increased injury rate.

    3. Some athletic shoes may increase performance on some surfaces, but also increase the risk of injury.

    4. There seems to be no connection of ACL size to injury rate.

    5. Situations that place a loaded knee joint in a combined position of flexion, valgus, and rotation of the tibia on the femur can rupture the ACL in a noncontact manner.

    6. Symptoms include hearing a pop, followed by rapid effusion, and a few minutes of nausea. The Lachman's maneuver or anterior drawer test, if done within five minutes of the injury, can test ligament integrity. Diagnosis by the athlete's physician and an MRI will confirm the diagnosis.

    7. Treatment includes splinting, icing compressive wrapping, the use of crutches, referral to a physician, and ultimately reconstructive surgery.

G. Posterior cruciate ligament (PCL) tears are less common than the ACL injuries. Most PCL injuries in athletics involve a fall on the flexed knee with the foot plantar flexed, resulting in the tibia striking the ground first and being pushed back.

    1. A positive sag test is diagnostic of a PCL tear.

    2. Treatment uses PRICE and assessment by the athlete's physician.

H. Meniscus tears involve the menisci of the knee, which help make a more concave surface for the condyles of the femur to rest and glide on. They can be torn when the knee is twisted suddenly and one or both menisci become trapped between the femur and tibia.

    1. Symptoms include slow swelling over several hours, pain, popping, locking, and giving way of the knee. Tibiofibular joint spaces may be tender.

    2. Treatment should include ice and compressive wrap, crutches, knee supports, and physician referral.

I. Epiphyseal growth-plate injuries are possible among immature athletes and can be serious to the growing athlete, so return to play should occur only with a physician's approval.

J. Osgood-Schlatter condition is a group of symptoms involving the tibial tubercle epiphysis, a small bump on the tibia where the patellar tendon attaches. It is a growth center and most likely affects males between the ages of 12 and 16 and females between 10 and 14 years of age.

   1. Symptoms include pain, swelling, weakness in the quadriceps, increased pain and swelling with activity, a visible lump, and pain when touched.

   2. Treatment involves prevention of progression, such as with a protective pad like a standard volleyball knee pad, a neoprene sleeve, ice every day after activities, anti-inflammatory medications, and stretching the hamstrings to alleviate pain. If the athlete continues to have increasing pain, he or she should return to the physician for further consultation.

K. Iliotibial band syndrome involves inflammation of the thick band of fibrous tissue that runs down the outside of the leg, beginning at the hip and extending to the outer side of the tibia, just below the knee.

   1. Symptoms include pain when the knee joint is moved, increasing with more movement.

   2. Treatment begins with analysis of the athlete's gait and training program to rule out mechanical problems or training errors, using proper footwear, icing, and stretching. Reduced activity will be necessary until symptoms subside.

L. Fractures around the knee are the result of high-energy trauma.

   1. A fracture of the patella could occur when the knee strikes a hard surface.

   2. Distal femoral and proximal tibial fractures may occur from violent twisting or falls from heights.

VOCABULARY REVIEW

Matching

Match the terms on the right with the definitions on the left. Terms may be used once, more than once, or not at all.

_____ 1. The point where the tibia meets with the femur

_____ 2. Swelling within the joint cavity

_____ 3. The point where the kneecap and femur are connected in the trochlear groove

_____ 4. Cartilage in the knee between the femoral condyle and the medial tibial plateau

_____ 5. The kneecap

_____ 6. Inward bending or twisting force

_____ 7. The growth plate at the end of bones

_____ 8. A ligament in the knee that attaches to the femur and the fibula allowing for stability in the knee joint

_____ 9. Cartilage in the knee between the lateral femoral condyle and the lateral tibial plateau

_____ 10. A ligament in the knee that attaches to the anterior aspect of the tibial plateau restricting anterior movement of the tibia on the femur

_____ 11. The thin layer of connective tissue over the ends of long bones

_____ 12. A ligament in the knee that attaches to the femur and tibia, allowing for stability in the knee joint

_____ 13. A grinding noise or sensation within a joint

_____ 14. The area of the attachment for the sartorius, gracilis, and semitendinosus to the anteriomedial tibia

_____ 15. A ligament in the knee that attaches to the posterior aspect of the tibial plateau, restricting posterior movement of the tibia on the femur

_____ 16. A large group of muscles in the front of the thigh

_____ 17. The back side of the patella that is covered with a thick layer of articular cartilage

_____ 18. A small bone, formed in a tendon, where it passes over a joint

_____ 19. A lubricating substance found in joints

_____ 20. The connective tissue that encompasses the patella and extends distally across the front of the knee

_____ 21. The rounded prominence found at the point of articulation with another bone

_____ 22. A double layer of connective tissue that lines joint cavities and produces synovial fluid

_____ 23. The top, flat portion of the tibia

A. anterior cruciate ligament (ACL)

B. articular cartilage

C. condyle

D. crepitus

E. effusion

F. epiphyseal plates

G. lateral collateral ligament (LCL)

H. lateral meniscus

I. medial collateral ligament

J. medial meniscus

K. patella

L. patellar tendon

M. patellofemoral joint

N. pes ansurine

O. posterior cruciate ligament (PCL)

P. quadriceps

Q. retropatellar surface

R. sesamoid

S. synovial fluid

T. synovial membrane

U. tibial plateau

V. tibiofemoral joint

W. valgus

X. varus

ANATOMY IDENTIFICATION

1. Label and color the structures of the knee.

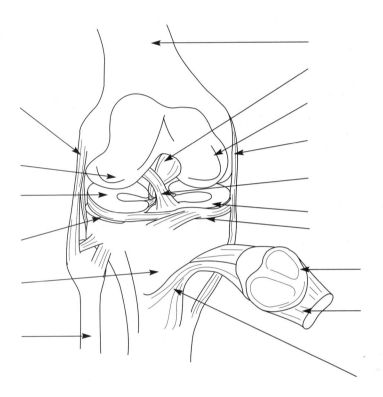

2. Label the following figure. Color the structures found at the ends of the femur and tibia.

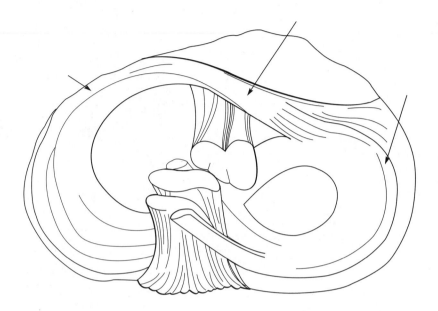

ACTIVITIES

1. Using a model of the knee joint that shows ligament and/or tendon attachments, identify all of the structures referred to in the textbook. Learn them well enough to be able to identify each when quizzed.

_____

_____

_____

_____

_____

2. Demonstrate the movements of the knee using the different muscles that control it. Use your knee or the knee of another person.

_____

_____

_____

_____

_____

ONLINE RESEARCH

■ Research current knee treatments on the Internet and describe how they differ from those described in the text.

_____

_____

_____

_____

_____

■ Find graphics of the knee on the Internet that show the structural relationships of the various bones, ligaments, tendons, muscles, and nerves of the knee. Draw a poster-sized representation of one of the graphics, focusing on knee anatomy. Be sure that all parts are labeled.

_____

_____

_____

_____

_____

CHAPTER 19

The Hip and Pelvis

KEY CONCEPTS

- The hip is the strongest joint in the human body. It allows a great deal of motion. The pelvis is a support structure for the body and transmits the weight of the axial skeleton to the lower limbs. The pelvis also provides points of attachment for many muscles, as well as providing protection for the organs of the digestive, urinary, and reproductive systems.

- The hip joint is where the spherical head of the femur fits into the deep socket of the pelvis. The ilium, sacrum, ischium, pubis, and coccyx are the structures that constitute the pelvis.

- Muscles from the lower back, pelvis, and thigh contribute to strength and stability. The largest muscle group of the hip and pelvic region is the gluteals. The adductor muscles assist in hip adduction. The quadriceps and hamstring muscles also assist in hip movement.

- In athletics, there are several common injuries to the hip and pelvic region.
  - Bursitis is inflammation of the bursae toward the outside of the hip. Treatment is to apply heat to the affected area and to stretch properly.
  - Fractures of the hip usually result from a fall and result in severe hip pain. Treatment will depend on the fracture type.
  - Quadriceps and hip flexor strains usually occur in athletes whose sports require repetitive sprinting, jumping, and kicking. Treatment consists of ice, compression and anti-inflammatory medications.
  - Hamstring strains result when these muscles are pulled too far too fast. Treatment is usually a combination of rest, ice, compression, and elevation with medication, and physical therapy.
  - Adductor strains usually result from sudden sideways changes in direction. Typically, they are difficult to treat; rest, ice, anti-inflammatory medications, and stretching are recommended.
  - Illiotibial band syndrome is an inflammation of the iliotibial band. Treatment includes analysis of gait and modifications of the athlete's training regimen.
  - Quadriceps contusions are the result of a direct blow to the thigh. Treatment consists of compression, ice, and protection from weight bearing.

(continues)

(continued)

- Myositis ossificans is a painful condition in which a calcium deposit forms within the muscle. Treatment involves heat, limitation of joint movement, and rehabilitative exercises.
- Iliac crest contusions are the result of a direct blow to the hip. Treatment involves ice and compression.
- Overuse injuries are the result of the cumulative effects of low-level stress on one particular area. Treatment may include a more well-rounded training routine.
- Stress fractures of the pelvis occur most often in runners and dancers. Treatment consists of rest and nonweight-bearing endurance exercises.

OUTLINE

I. The Hip and Pelvis

  A. The hip, one of the most stable joints in the body, is a freely movable, ball-and-socket joint that lies between the head of the femur and the acetabulum of the pelvis.

    1. Most hip injuries result from the smaller muscles of the hip being overused or pushed too hard.

    2. The function of the pelvis is to transmit weight from the axial skeleton to the lower limbs when standing or to the ischial tuberosities when sitting.

    3. The pelvis provides attachments for various muscles, houses parts of the digestive, urinary, and reproductive systems.

    4. The female bone structure is slightly less dense than the male's, and it is smaller, shorter, and wider. Also bone protrusions for muscle attachment are not as sharply defined.

  B. Skeletal structure

    1. The ilium is a broad, flared portion that constitutes the upper and lateral sections of the pelvis, with the iliac crest as the upper ridge.

      a. The greater sciatic notch allows the sciatic nerve to pass through to the leg below.

      b. The iliac fossa helps create a basin for the lower abdominal organs.

    2. The sacrum is composed of five fused vertebrae and connects directly to the ilium.

    3. The ischium bears weight when sitting and is attached to the pubis in front and to the ilium laterally and to the back. The large opening in the ischium is the obturator foramina, where blood vessels and nerves pass into the legs.

    4. The pubis makes up the front of the pelvic bones and is located in front and below the bladder. The center of the pubis is the pubic symphysis, where the two sides of the pubis fuse.

    5. The coccyx (tailbone) is composed of three to five rudimentary vertebrae and is connected to the lower portion of the sacrum. It is extremely susceptible to shock fracture, as might be induced from a fall, and may cause damage to several nearby nerve pathways.

C. Primary muscles of the pelvis, hip, and thigh

1. The gluteal muscles provide the largest group. The gluteus medius, gluteus minimus, and gluteus maximus assist in hip extension, internal and external rotation, and abduction.

2. Muscles that assist in hip flexion (hip flexors) include the iliopsoas, sartorius, pectineus, and rectus femoris.

3. The hip adductor group includes the adductor longus, adductor brevis, and adductor magnus.

4. The quadriceps (vastus medialis, vastus intermedius, vastus lateralis, and rectus femoris) cause hip flexion.

5. The hamstrings (biceps femoris, semitendinosus, and semimembranosus) cause hip extension.

II. Common Injuries and Conditions of the Hip and Thigh

A. Bursitis is most commonly located over the outside of the hip (trochanteric bursitis), especially among athletes who do not sufficiently stretch and warm up in this area.

1. Symptoms include tenderness over the outer portion of the hip, which can be made worse by walking, running, or twisting the hip.

2. Initially the condition is treated with heat, followed by stretching exercises and ice massage. Nonsteroidal anti-inflammatory medicines are also helpful.

B. A hip fracture refers to a break in the proximal portion of the femur, most commonly femoral neck fractures, intertrochanteric fractures, or subtrochanteric fractures. In young patients, extreme trauma, as in automobile accidents, is usually necessary for a hip fracture.

1. Symptoms include severe hip pain, an abnormally rotated leg, and increased pain with movement.

2. Treatments vary and must be discussed with the surgeon.

C. Quadriceps and hip flexor strains are common in sports requiring jumping, kicking, or repetitive sprinting.

1. Most quadriceps strains involve the rectus femoris and/or the iliopsoas muscles.

2. Treatment includes icing, compression with an elastic wrap, and anti-inflammatory medications. Rehabilitation should be progressive and sport-specific.

D. Hamstring strains most frequently affect the long head of the biceps femoris and can range from microtears in a small area to a complete tear in the muscle or its tendons, usually called a hamstring tear.

1. Hamstring strains may be due to insufficiently warming up, developing the quadriceps more than the hamstrings, inflexibility, or a direct blow to the back of the leg.

2. Symptoms include sharp pain in the back of the thigh, bruising, swelling, loss of strength in the upper leg.

3. Nonsurgical treatment usually can heal hamstring strains. A combination of RICE (rest, ice, compression, and elevation), medication, and physical therapy, with pain relief coming from aspirin or ibuprofen is often enough. Crutches and massage may also be recommended.

4. Rehabilitation should begin soon after the injury, progressing into a weight-training program focused on balancing strength between the hamstrings and quadriceps.

E. Adductor (groin) strains are common in sports requiring sideways changes in direction, most involving the adductor longus.

    1. Most strains are grade I or II, characterized by groin pain when running or kicking.

    2. Treatment is difficult and the risk of reinjury is high. Rest, ice, anti-inflammatory medications followed by adductor stretching and strengthening is a usual approach.

F. Iliotibial band syndrome involves inflammation of the thick band of fibrous tissue that runs down the outside of the leg, beginning at the hip and extending to the outer side of the tibia just below the knee.

    1. Symptoms include irritation and pain when the knee joint is moved, increasing with more movement.

    2. Treatment begins with analysis of the athlete's gait and training program to rule out mechanical problems or training errors, using proper footwear, icing, and stretching. Reduced activity will be necessary until symptoms subside.

G. Quadriceps contusions are common in football, rugby, soccer, and basketball, usually caused by a direct blow to the thigh from a helmet or knee.

    1. The injury may limit motion and affect gait, with the severity of the contusion graded by the range of motion in the hip when evaluated.

    2. Treatment includes immediate compression, ice, and use of crutches. Massage may cause more damage and is contraindicated.

H. Myositis ossificans is a very painful condition in which an ossifying mass may form within the muscle, usually the result of recurrent trauma to a quadriceps muscle that was not properly protected after the initial injury.

    1. Symptoms include a hard, painful mass in the soft tissue of the thigh, loss of knee bending motion. It is ultimately diagnosed with x-ray at least four weeks after injury.

    2. Early treatment is with heat, limitation of joint motion, and rehabilitative exercises. Passive stretching and vigorous exercise for the first six months is discouraged. Surgical excision may be necessary if pain and limited motion persist beyond one year.

I. An iliac crest contusion, or hip pointer, is a very painful injury caused by a direct blow to the hip.

    1. Symptoms include extreme tenderness, swelling, and eccymosis over the iliac crest.

    2. Treatment includes application of ice and compression.

J. Overuse injuries are common among one-sport athletes, caused by cumulative effects of very low levels of stress.

    1. Examples include chronic muscle strains, stress fractures, tendonitis, snapping hip, and bursitis.

    2. Athletes with these problems should rest from the sport and use cross-training techniques.

K. Stress fractures of the pelvis occur most often in runners and dancers. Femur stress fractures are common in runners.

    1. Symptoms include chronic, ill-defined pain over the groin and thigh. If symptoms do not resolve with rest and rehabilitative exercise, the athlete should be examined by a sports medicine specialist using x-rays and bone scans.

    2. Treatment includes rest and nonweight-bearing endurance exercises, such as running in water or swimming.

VOCABULARY REVIEW

Matching

Match the terms on the right with the definitions on the left. Terms may be used once, more than once, or not at all.

_____ 1. A broad, flared bone that makes up the upper and lateral sections of the pelvis

_____ 2. The portion of the vertebral column between the lumbar vertebrae and the coccyx; it bears the weight of the body when sitting

_____ 3. A group of muscles that extend the hip and flex the knee; consists of the biceps femoris, semitendinosus, and semimembranosus

_____ 4. A painful injury caused by a direct blow to the hip, resulting in ecchymosis, tenderness, and swelling; also known as the hip pointer

_____ 5. A muscle group that aids in the adduction of the hip

_____ 6. The bone in the pelvis to the front of and below the bladder

_____ 7. Inflammation of the iliotibial band

_____ 8. The tailbone

_____ 9. A muscle group that consists of the adductor longus, adductor brevis, and adductor magnus

_____ 10. A space in the pelvis through which the sciatic nerve travels to the legs

_____ 11. A painful condition in which a calcium deposit forms within the muscle

_____ 12. The portion of the pelvis that is attached to the pubis in front and the ilium laterally in the back; it bears the weight of the body when sitting

_____ 13. The large openings in the ischium through which blood vessels and nerves pass to the legs

_____ 14. A muscle group that aids in the flexion of the hip

_____ 15. The upper ridge of the ilium

_____ 16. The center of the pubis where the two sides of the pubis are fused together

_____ 17. It consists of the iliopsoas, sartorius, pectineus, and rectus femoris

A. adductor muscles

B. coccyx

C. greater sciatic notch

D. hamstring muscles

E. hip flexors

F. iliac crest

G. iliac crest contusion

H. iliac fossa

I. iliotibial band syndrome

J. ilium

K. ischium

L. myositis ossificans

M. obturator foramina

N. pubis

O. sacrum

P. symphysis

ANATOMY IDENTIFICATION

1. For the following pelvis diagrams, label all structures referred to in the textbook. Color the three bones of the pelvis three different colors.

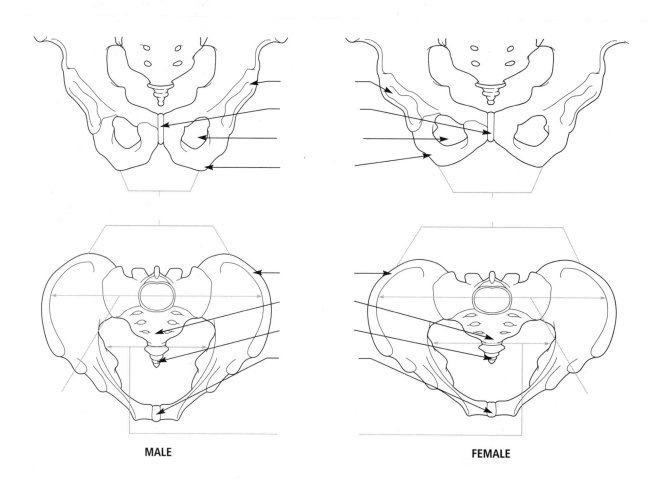

MALE   FEMALE

2. Label and color each of the muscles of the leg. Use different shades of the same color for the hamstrings and different shades of another color for the quadriceps (for example, different shades of red for the hamstrings, different shades of green for the quadriceps, and then colors other than red or green for the rest of the muscles). If the same muscle appears on both views of the leg, be sure to color it the same color on both.

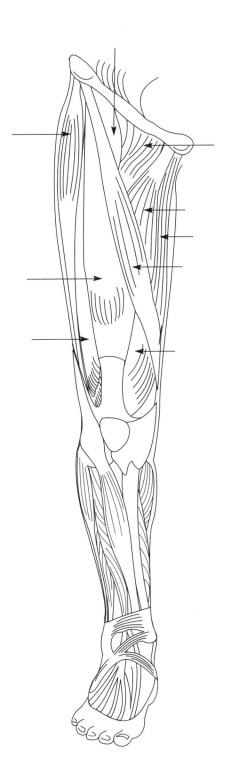
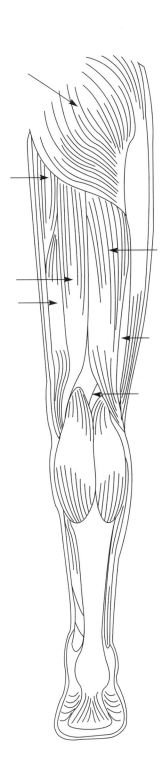

ACTIVITIES

1. Look at a model of a hip joint that shows ligament and/or tendon connections. Identify each structure referred to in the textbook. Then teach someone else about the hip structure without looking at notes, diagrams, or other reference materials.

_____

_____

_____

_____

2. Practice demonstrating the actions of each muscle of the hip, using your own leg and hip.

_____

_____

_____

_____

3. Of all the bone groups in the body, the pelvis bones demonstrate the most differences in structure between males and females. Examine the model of male and female pelvic bones, and be able to identify those areas that differ.

_____

_____

_____

_____

ONLINE RESEARCH

■ Research current or alternative techniques for treating hip joint injuries. Describe how they differ from what is discussed in the textbook.

_____

_____

_____

_____

■ According to the textbook, the hip joint is very strong and stable. Research the common hip injuries, both athletic and nonathletic.

_____

_____

_____

_____

CHAPTER 20

The Elbow, Wrist, and Hand

KEY CONCEPTS

- The humerus articulates with the radius and ulna, forming a hinge joint. Ligaments, nerves, and muscles aid in movement of the elbow.
- The hand, including the wrist, consists of 27 bones. The carpals are the 8 bones that make up the wrist. The 5 metacarpals form the structure of the hand. The 14 phalanges are the bones of the fingers.
- Common injuries of the elbow include:
  - Contusions, the result of force applied to the bony prominences of the elbow. Treatment consists of rest, ice, compression, and elevation.
  - Olecranon bursitis, which is inflammation of the bursa. Treatment depends on the presence of infection. If the bursa is not infected, the bursitis can be treated with ice, rest, and anti-inflammatory pain medications.
  - Ulnar nerve contusion, or hitting the funny bone, which results from a direct blow to the ulnar nerve. Treatment is usually not necessary, as this generally subsides on its own.
  - Elbow strains, which result from stress being placed on the elbow. Treatment is aimed at prevention through proper technique, use of appropriate equipment, and limitation of stress on the joint.
  - Elbow sprains, which result from forced hyperextension by side-to-side forces on the joint. The treatment is similar to that for strains; some commercial braces may help.
  - Elbow dislocations, which result from bones in the joint being displaced. The athlete must be transported to the nearest medical facility.
  - Fractures of the elbow and forearm, resulting from forces that crack and break the bony structures. Treatment involves immobilization, ice, elevation, and prompt referral to a physician.
  - Volkmann's contracture, a serious condition that results from a lack of blood flow to the forearm.
  - Nerve injuries, which can occur to the ulnar, radial, or medial nerve.
- Common injuries to the wrist and hand include:
  - Fractures, resulting from excessive force to the bony structure of the hand and wrist. Treatment includes ice, immobilization, and immediate treatment by a physician.

(continues)

(continued)

- Contusions, which result from force or a fall onto a hard surface.
- Sprains, resulting from forces that place stress on the joints and cause ligament damage.
- Tendonitis, an inflammation of the tendons in the wrist and fingers.
- Nerve damage, which can occur to the nerves in the hand and fingers as a result of repetitive stresses on the hand and wrist. Treatment should include rest, and icing may provide some relief.
- Ganglion cysts are a small, hard lumps above a tendon that encloses a joint. If the cyst is painless, treatment is not necessary.
- Boutonniére deformity, an injury to the extensor tendon that affects two joints of the finger. After this injury, treatment is effective for only a limited period of time.

OUTLINE

I. The Elbow, Wrist, and Hand

    A. The wrist and hand are made up of 27 bones.

        1. The eight bones that make up the wrist are called the carpals.

        2. The five metacarpals form the structure of the hand.

        3. There are 14 total phalanges bones: two for the thumb, three for each of the other four fingers.

II. The Elbow

    A. The three bones of the elbow joint are the humerus in the upper arm and the radius and ulna in the lower arm.

    B. Many ligaments, nerves, muscles, bursa sacs surround the elbow joint.

    C. Muscles of the elbow that flex the forearm include the brachialis, the biceps brachii, and the brachioradialis; two muscles that extend the arm are the triceps brachii and the anconeus.

III. Common Injuries of the Elbow

    A. Contusions are common and may involve the muscles of the forearm and subcutaneous bony prominences of the elbow. Direct blows to these muscular areas can result in bruising and subsequent bleeding, producing stiffness during function and active range of motion.

        1. The area must be protected against additional trauma and to guard against the possible development of myositis ossificans.

        2. Treatment includes rest, ice, compression, and elevation (RICE).

    B. Olecranon bursitis can be accompanied by infection due to the frequent abrasions that occur over the tip of the elbow.

        1. Uninfected bursitis is treated with ice compresses, rest, anti-inflammatory and pain medications.

        2. Occasionally, aspiration of the bursa fluid is necessary—a procedure that can be performed in a doctor's office.

C. Ulnar nerve contusion, due to a direct blow to the medial epicondyle of the humerus causes immediate pain and a burning sensation shooting down the ulnar side of the forearm to the ring and little fingers (otherwise known as hitting the "funny bone"). No treatment is usually necessary.

D. Strains to the elbow normally occur as a result of the tremendous stresses being placed on the elbow joint, especially in sports requiring throwing or swimming motions.

　　1. Acute strains occur with a sudden overload to the elbow joint. Symptoms include the history of an incident of sudden, excessive overload followed by tenderness over the affected area and pain on function or resisted motion.

　　2. Chronic strains are the result of continued overuse. Continued trauma in this area can develop into overuse syndromes and chronic degenerative processes.

　　3. The most common areas of acute strains are the common flexor tendon around the medial epicondyle and the common extensor tendon around the lateral epicondyle.

E. Epicondylitis occurs in the region of the medial and lateral epicondyle of the humerus, usually caused by repeated overload of the attached musculotendinous units; sometimes called tennis elbow.

　　1. If the condition occurs in young athletes; for example, little league elbow, it can be accompanied by or due to injury to the growth plates of the epiphysis.

　　2. Symptoms include pain when used, possible swelling, local tenderness, and pain with resisted wrist motion.

　　3. Without proper treatment, the condition may develop into prolonged degenerative changes, resulting in chronic epicondylitis, contractures of the elbow, reduced friction, and possible rupture of the muscle tendon unit.

　　4. Preventative measures include using proper technique and equipment, limiting stress, adequately warming up, and stretching.

　　5. Treatment includes rest, ice, compression and elevation (RICE), and modifying activities that aggravate the condition.

F. Sprains of the elbow are usually due to forced hyperextension or valgus/varus (side-to-side) forces.

　　1. Symptoms include hearing a click or pop along with sharp pain at the time of the injury, tenderness, localized swelling, and pain when trying to repeat the mechanism of injury. Pain is usually relieved by bending the elbow.

　　2. Treatment is the same as with strains.

G. Dislocation of the elbow most commonly involves the posterior displacement of the ulna and radius in relationship to the humerus; often the result of a fall onto an outstretched hand with the elbow in extension.

　　1. Symptoms include observing an obvious deformity, loss of elbow function, and considerable pain. The initial examination must include an evaluation of the circulation and nerve function of the hands and fingers.

　　2. All elbow dislocations should be properly immobilized and referred to a physician immediately. Transport to the athlete's physician or the nearest medical facility is critical because of possible vascular and neurological damage.

H. Fractures of the elbow and forearm are usually the result of either direct trauma or indirect stresses transmitted through the upper extremity as the result of falling on an outstretched arm. Many fractures in younger athletes involve the epiphyseal growth plates.

    1. Symptoms are directly related to the degree of severity. Point tenderness is common, accompanied by varying amounts of hemorrhaging or swelling. There may also be limited range of motion, disability at the elbow or hand, and an increase in pain with attempted movements.

    2. Treatment involves immobilization, ice, elevation, and prompt referral to a physician or medical clinic. Serious elbow fractures must be treated as a medical emergency.

I. Volkmann's contracture occurs in the absence of blood flow (ischemia) to the forearm. This can be caused by increased pressure from swelling, trauma, or fracture, and can lead to contracture, where the joint remains bent and cannot straighten.

    1. There are three levels of severity in Volkmann's contracture:

        a. Mild involves flexion contracture of two or three fingers, with no limited loss of sensation.

        b. Moderate involves all fingers being flexed and the thumb stuck in the palm. The wrist may be stuck in flexion, and there is usually some loss of sensation in the hand.

        c. Severe involves all muscles in the forearm that both flex and extend the wrist and fingers, a severely disabling condition.

    2. Symptoms include severe pain when a muscle running through a compartment is passively moved; the forearm may be swollen, shiny, and painful when squeezed. Pain does not improve with rest, but continues to worsen with time. If the condition is not corrected, there will be decreased sensation, weakness, and paleness of the skin.

J. Injury to the ulnar nerve can involve irritation, compression, or entrapment in the cubital tunnel (cubital tunnel syndrome). Symptoms include pain along the inner aspect of the elbow, tenderness over the medial epicondylar groove, and paresthesia (numbness or tingling) in the ring finger and little finger.

K. Injury to the radial nerve, which passes through a tunnel formed by several muscles and tendons, includes entrapment (radial tunnel syndrome). Symptoms include pain over the lateral aspect of the elbow and may be present over the anterior radial head.

L. Injury to the median nerve includes entrapment or compression due to hypertrophy of the pronator teres or repetitive pronation of the forearm (pronator teres syndrome). Symptoms include pain radiating down the anterior forearm, with numbness and tingling in the thumb, index, and middle fingers. Resistive pronation may increase the pain.

IV. Hand and Wrist Injuries

A. The eight bones that make up the wrist are known as carpals; the metacarpals form the structure of the hand, and the phalanges the fingers.

B. Muscles of the hand and wrist includes two flexor carpi muscles that flex the wrist and the three extensor carpi muscles that extend the wrist with the assistance of the extensor digitorum communis.

C. Hand and wrist injuries common to athletes include fractures, dislocations, contusions, sprains, tendonitis, and nerve impingements.

D. Many types of fractures to the wrist and hand are possible.

1. Finger fractures can involve any of the 14 phalanges bones. Most can be treated with a finger splint.

2. Boxer's fracture is a break of the fifth metacarpal leading to the little finger.

3. Baseball (mallet) finger is a painful injury that occurs when a ball or other object strikes the tip of the finger, bending it down beyond its normal range of motion, which tears the finger tendon and damages cartilage.

4. Jersey finger is caused by tearing the flexor tendon to the fingertip, which usually occurs from grabbing a jersey during a tackle. The ring finger is most often affected.

5. A scaphoid fracture affects the scaphoid bone, one of the wrist's carpal bones. Palpation of the anatomical snuffbox will cause pain, indicating that a fracture may be present.

6. Colles fracture is a break of the radius just above the wrist.

7. Treatment, as with all fractures, includes rest, ice, compression, elevation, support (RICES), and evaluation by a physician.

E. Dislocations and subluxations of the hand and wrist are fairly common, such as a ball striking the fingertips or a finger getting hooked into a piece of equipment (like a football helmet).

   1. Symptoms include immediate pain and swelling, and a crooked finger, which usually cannot be bent or straightened.

   2. Treatment includes ice, immobilization, and immediate treatment by a physician.

F. Contusions are usually caused by direct blows or falling onto a hard surface. When the nail becomes contused, pressure may require a physician to drain blood from beneath the nail.

G. Sprains of the wrist and hand are injuries to the ligaments and were dealt with in Chapter 16.

   1. Gamekeeper's thumb is a sprain of the ulnar collateral ligament of the metacarpalphalangeal joint (MPJ), which is common in alpine skiing, where a force is applied to the medial side of the thumb, forcing the MPJ to stretch, tear, or even rupture.

H. Tendonitis is the inflammation of tendons caused by overuse or repetitive stress.

   1. Symptoms include ache or pain at the wrist, which worsens with forceful gripping, rapid wrist movements, or moving the wrist or fingers to an extreme position.

   2. Treatment is the same as any other tendonitis.

   3. One of the most common sites in the wrist for problems is at the base of the thumb near the anatomical snuffbox (deQuervain's tenosynovitis).

I. Nerve impingement (carpal tunnel syndrome) is an inflammatory disorder caused by repetitive stress, physical injury, or other conditions that cause swelling around the median nerve near the carpal tunnel.

   1. Symptoms include pain, numbness, and tingling in the wrist, hand, and fingers (except the little finger). There is also a tendency to drop things, loss of the sense of heat or cold, and a swollen feeling even though it is not visibly swollen. Symptoms may occur only when the hand is being used or only when at rest.

   2. Treatment includes rest, ice, and in severe cases surgery to decompress the median nerve.

J. A ganglion cyst is a small, usually hard lump above a tendon or in a capsule that encloses a joint; also called a synovial hernia or synovial cyst. It is common in handball, racquetball, squash, and tennis.

K. The boutonnière deformity is an extensor tendon injury affecting the proximal interphalangeal (PIP) joint at the middle of the finger or the distal interphalangeal (DIP) joint at the end of the finger.

   1. Symptoms include problems flexing and extending the finger; a physician should be contacted immediately. The finger joints will be painful and tender, the finger misshapen, and the athlete will not be able to straighten it.

   2. Treatment must be done promptly, or the athlete may not regain normal use of the finger.

VOCABULARY REVIEW

Matching

Match the terms on the right with the definitions on the left. Terms may be used once, more than once, or not at all.

_____ 1. Tendonitis originating in the base of the thumb, on the back side of the wrist, and the palm side of the wrist

_____ 2. A chronic strain of the medial or lateral epicondyle in the elbow; often known as tennis elbow

_____ 3. Injury to the thumb that results in tearing or stretching of the MP joint or rupture of the ulnar collateral ligament

_____ 4. The abnormal movement of one of the bones that constitute a joint

_____ 5. Inflammation of tendons caused by overuse or repetitive motions

_____ 6. A tear of the extensor tendon of the PIP joint, at the middle of the finger, and the DIP joint that controls the fingertip

_____ 7. An inflammatory disorder caused by irritation of the tissues and nerves around the medial nerve

_____ 8. Irritation, compression, and entrapment of the ulnar nerve

_____ 9. Entrapment of the radial nerve

_____ 10. A break in the scaphoid bone in the thumb

_____ 11. An injury to the finger resulting from tearing of the finger tendon and damaging the cartilage

A. boutonnière deformity
B. carpal tunnel syndrome
C. cubital tunnel syndrome
D. deQuervain's tenosynovitis
E. epicondylitis
F. gamekeeper's thumb
G. ganglion
H. jersey finger
I. lateral epicondyle
J. baseball (mallet) finger
K. medial epicondyle
L. median nerve
M. olecranon bursitis
N. pronator teres syndrome
O. radial nerve
P. radial tunnel syndrome
Q. scaphoid fracture
R. subluxation
S. tendonitis
T. tennis elbow
U. ulnar nerve
V. Volkmann's contracture

_____ 12. A nerve within the brachial plexus that passes through the cubital tunnel in the posterior aspect of the medial epicondyle

_____ 13. A small, hard lump above a tendon or in the capsule that encloses a joint

_____ 14. An injury to the finger resulting in tearing of the flexor tendon in the fingertip

_____ 15. The bony end of the humerus that lies to the outside of the elbow joint

_____ 16. A condition in which the muscles in the palm side of the forearm shorten, causing the fingers to form a fist and the wrist to bend

_____ 17. The bony end of the humerus that forms with the elbow joint

_____ 18. A nerve within the brachial plexus that crosses the anterior elbow, passes between the heads of the pronator teres, and runs distal to the joint

_____ 19. Inflammation of the bursa over the olecranon process of the elbow

_____ 20. A chronic strain of the lateral epicondyle in the elbow; often known as epicondylitis

_____ 21. Entrapment or compression of the median nerve

_____ 22. A nerve within the brachial plexus that passes anteriorly to the lateral epicondyle and lies in a tunnel of several muscles and tendons

Crossword Puzzle

Identify the terms described in the puzzle clues, then write the letters in the boxes. (Many terms are more than one word.)

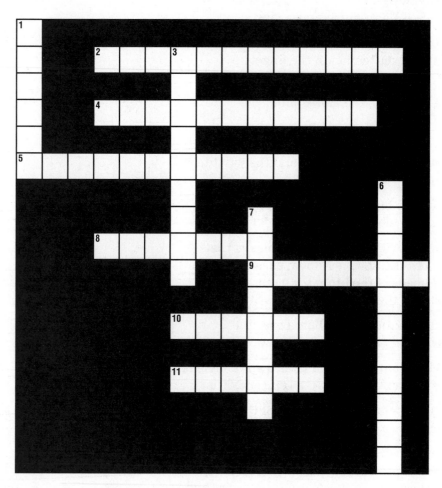

Across

  2. a passageway from the forearm through the wrist _____

  4. hand bones _____

  5. abnormal movement of one of the bones of a joint _____

  8. upper arm bone _____

  9. wrist bones _____

 10. a fracture in the fifth metacarpal _____

 11. a nerve that lies in a tunnel of several muscles and tendons _____

Down

  1. bone on the thumb side of the forearm _____

  3. finger bones _____

  6. displacement of a bone from its normal position _____

  7. decreased blood supply to an organ or tissue _____

ANATOMY IDENTIFICATION

1. Label and color the hand and wrist bones. Label the groups of the bones indicated by the brackets.

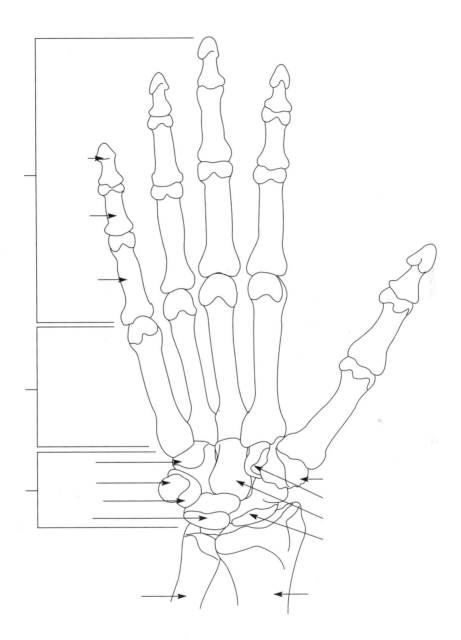

2. Label and color the elbow structures. Using a bracket, identify the ulnar collateral ligament.

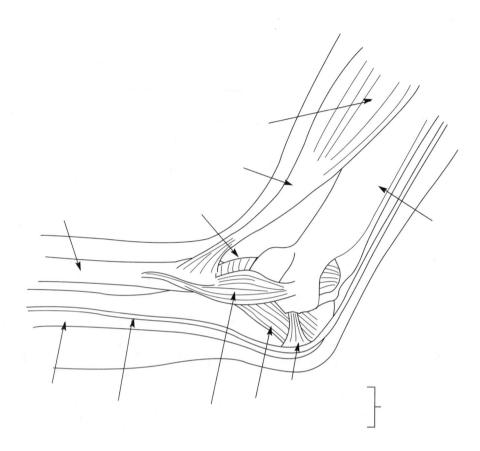

ACTIVITIES

1. Study models of the wrist and elbow, identifying all structures, including parts of the bones referred to in the textbook. Be able to identify these structures when quizzed.

_____

_____

_____

_____

_____

2. Practice demonstrating the wrist and elbow movements described in the textbook, using your own elbow and wrist.

_____

_____

_____

_____

_____

ONLINE RESEARCH

■ Research current and alternative treatments for one of the disorders described in the textbook. Discuss any recent discoveries about the disorder that have resulted in a modification of the disorder's treatment?

_____

_____

_____

_____

_____

CHAPTER 21

The Shoulder

KEY CONCEPTS

- Three joints make up the shoulder girdle: the sternoclavicular joint, the acromioclavicular joint, and the glenohumeral joint.
- The four muscles that make up the rotator cuff are the subscapularis, the supraspinatus, the infraspinatus, and the teres minor.
- The stability of the shoulder is maintained by the combined effort of the deltoid muscle and the rotator-cuff muscles. This is called a force couple: two equal forces acting in opposite directions to rotate the bones of the shoulder girdle around an axis.
- The shoulder complex is made up of three joints. Movement of the shoulder complex occurs with the aid of ligaments, cartilage, and layers of muscles. Stability of the shoulder complex results from the coordinated movements of the scapula and humerus. This is the most mobile of the upper extremity joints.
- Injuries to the shoulder result from overuse or trauma. Common overuse injuries include:
  - Impingement syndrome, resulting from narrowing of the space between the humeral head and the acromion. Treatment for this injury usually involves correction of improper technique, preseason conditioning, and specialized taping.
  - Rotator-cuff tears, in which there is damage to the muscles that make up the rotator cuff. There can be varying degrees of tears; treatment depends on the severity of the tear.
  - Muscle strains, which usually resolve within a few days. Immediate treatment is with PRICE.
  - Biceps tendonitis, an inflammation of the tendon that lies adjacent to the rotator cuff.
  - Biceps tendon rupture, the tearing away of the tendon from its point of attachment.
- Traumatic injuries to the shoulder include:
  - Anterior shoulder dislocation, in which the head of the humerus comes out of the socket. Immediate treatment by a physician should be sought.
  - Glenoid labrum injuries, which can occur with a shoulder dislocation. Structures in the glenoid fossa are torn or damaged. Treatment for mild injuries includes strengthening the area. For more involved injuries, surgery may be required.

(continues)

165

(continued)

- Multidirectional instabilities, which are injuries that occur when the joint slips out of place with little or no force. Weight training to strengthen the area is often helpful.
- Acromioclavicular separations, which result from a direct blow to the tip of the shoulder. An athlete with this injury should be seen by a physician. There are varying degrees of sprain with this injury.
- Injury to the brachial plexus, which results in pain and is caused by a blow to the head and neck that stretches the nerves on the opposite side. Treatment may include rest, ice packs, anti-inflammatory medication, and strengthening exercises.
- Shoulder fractures, which are breaks to any of the bones in the shoulder complex. Treatment should be sought from a physician.

OUTLINE

I. The Shoulder Girdle Complex
   A. Structure and function
      1. Dynamic stability refers to mobility along with stability, which the shoulder accomplishes through the coordinated movements of the scapula in concert with the humerus.
      2. The head of the humerus is attached to the glenoid fossa of the scapula to make up the glenohumeral joint, which is supported with numerous muscles, ligaments, and soft tissue. At the same time the shallowness of the socket allows for a great deal of movement.
      3. The acromion process is superior to the glenohumeral joint, forming the acromioclavicular (AC) joint with the clavicle. The other end of the clavicle is attached to the sternum to form the sternoclavicular (SC) joint.
      4. The scapulothoracic joint is not a true joint, but allows the scapula to slide over the back side of the thorax. Its stability comes entirely from muscle action.
      5. Several muscle groups working together synergistically are responsible for dynamic stability of the shoulder.
   B. The rotator cuff is a set of four deep muscles of the glenohumeral joint, which arise from the scapula and insert onto the superior aspect of the humerus.
      1. The subscapularis inserts onto the humerus anteriorly.
      2. The supraspinatus inserts onto the humerus anteriosuperiorly.
      3. The infraspinatus inserts onto the humerus posterosuperiorly.
      4. The teres minor inserts onto the humerus posteriorly.
   C. A muscle force couple is formed by the actions of the deltoid and rotator cuff muscles, allowing the humeral head to spin, while remaining in place on the glenoid.
   D. Scapulothoracic mechanics, allowing the scapula to move in several different planes, are accomplished by using the upper, middle, and lower trapezius, rhomboids, serratus anterior, and pectoralis minor muscles.
II. Overuse Injuries to the Shoulder
   A. Overuse injuries are usually limited to soft tissues.

B. Impingement syndrome describes a situation causing injury when the space between the humeral head and acromion becomes narrowed. The bones "impinge," or squeeze, structures within that space. Structures affected are the joint capsule, tendons of the rotator cuff, and a bursa.

    1. Impingement causes mechanical irritation of the cuff tendons, resulting in hemorrhage and swelling, commonly called tendonitis of the rotator cuff.

    2. If the bursa is involved, bursitis is the result.

    3. Symptoms include pain and tenderness in the glenohumeral area, pain and/or weakness with abduction in mid-range, limited internal rotation, positive results from special tests like the Hawkin's impingement test, and tenderness to palpation in the subacromial area.

    4. Treatment involves correction of improper sport technique, preseason conditioning, and specialized taping.

C. Rotator-cuff tears may be partial or full thickness.

    1. Symptoms include pain, with the arm still able to move in a normal range of motion for partial tears. With complete tears normal range of motion is not possible, the athlete is unable to lift the arm overhead, and when individuals attempt to, the shoulder can be observed to shrug or hike.

    2. Small and partial thickness tears may respond to a shoulder rehabilitation program. Most moderate to large tears (and small tears that do not respond to rehabilitation) require surgery.

D. Muscle strains can be caused by overuse or traumatic injury.

    1. Symptoms include pain and tenderness in the muscle belly, provoked by direct palpation, stretch, and contraction against resistance. There may be a delay of a day or two before symptoms show up (delayed onset of muscle soreness or DOMS).

    2. Treatment includes PRICE (protection, rest, ice, compression, and elevation), gentle stretching, and a strengthening program.

E. Biceps (long head) tendonitis can cause discomfort in the front of the shoulder and may be confused with rotator-cuff tendonitis. Both can be caused by impingement and are treated the same way.

F. Biceps tendon rupture results in a sudden onset of pain of the shoulder, associated with a pop sound during vigorous activity.

    1. Symptoms include drooping of the biceps near the distal upper arm, ecchymoses in the upper arm.

    2. Treatment does not always involve surgery. Protection, rest, and ice in the acute stage, with a gradual return to strengthening and sport activity over a few weeks, is usually the treatment of choice.

III. Traumatic Shoulder Injuries

A. Anterior shoulder dislocation of the glenohumeral joint results in the head of the humerus being completely out of the glenoid fossa, most commonly anteroinferiorly (front and down).

    1. The injury requires immediate transport to a physician, who will also check for other injuries such as fractures, glenoid labial tears, and axillary nerve damage.

    2. A Hills-Sach lesion can occur if the head of the humerus hits the front of the glenoid hard enough to cause an indentation.

    3. If the initial injury is not properly managed and fully rehabilitated, there is a high risk for recurrent dislocations. Immobilization may be as long as eight weeks.

B. Glenoid labrum injuries involve the deepest soft tissues in the shoulder, and can occur along with dislocation. Baseball pitchers are susceptible to degenerative changes in the labrum causing it to become loose, permitting the humeral head to slip forward.

   1. Symptoms include pain and a popping sensation, resulting in limited use of the arm, with varying degrees of weakness. Special tests and an MRI will help with an accurate diagnosis.

   2. Treatment includes a guided strengthening program. Suspected labial tears must be referred to a physician.

C. Multidirectional instabilities refer to the ability of the athlete to voluntarily dislocate his or her shoulders, usually creating problems with overhead sports. Weight-bearing exercises are often helpful.

D. Acromioclavicular separation is a traumatic sprain of the AC joint, usually from a direct blow to the tip of the shoulder.

   1. Symptoms include pain near the AC joint and evidence of deformity.

   2. Treatment involves physician referral. First-degree sprains may be treated with PRICE. Second- and third-degree sprains often require three to eight weeks of immobilization.

E. Brachial plexus injury, often called a stinger or burner, is caused by a stretching of the brachial plexus on the opposite side.

   1. Symptoms include intense pain from the neck down to the arm and an on-fire or pins-and-needles sensation; the arm may also be weak and numb.

   2. Treatment involves referral to a sports medicine specialist, rest, ice pack on the neck, anti-inflammatory medication, and strengthening exercises for the neck and shoulders.

   3. Prevention includes keeping the neck and shoulder muscles as strong as possible, wearing properly fitted equipment that distributes collision forces, and using proper technique.

F. Fractures of the shoulder commonly include the clavicle and humerus. Scapular fractures may not be seen on standard x-rays but are present on bone scans. Suspected bone fractures should be supported and the athlete taken to an emergency room.

IV. Is It a Shoulder Injury?

A. Pain in the shoulder region does not always indicate a shoulder problem.

B. Cardiac problems can be referred pain to the left shoulder, neck, and arm.

C. A spleen injury can refer pain to the left shoulder and down the upper portion of the left arm (Kehr's sign).

V. Additional Stretching and Strengthening Exercises for the Shoulder

VOCABULARY REVIEW

Crossword Puzzle

Identify the terms described in the puzzle clues, then write the letters in the boxes. (Many terms are more than one word.)

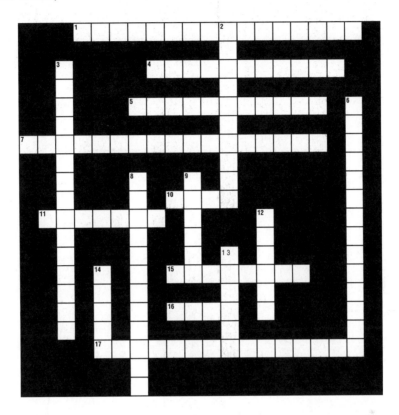

Across

1. mobility with steadiness _____
4. when space between the humeral head and acromion becomes narrowed _____
5. the four muscles of the glenohumeral joint _____
7. AC _____
10. muscle soreness that appears one or two days after the injury (abbr.) _____
11. burner _____
15. a kind of pain that occurs somewhere other than where the damage is _____
16. upper portion of the humerus _____
17. anterior projection of the scapula _____

Down

2. inflammation of the tissue connecting muscles to bones _____
3. muscles that act together to enhance joint movement _____
6. a group of nerves passing into the shoulder _____
8. synovial ball and socket joint of the shoulder _____
9. two forces in opposite directions that cause rotation _____
12. the deepest soft tissues in the shoulder _____
13. tissue that connects the biceps to the shoulder girdle _____
14. a slightly concave projection of the scapula _____

ANATOMY IDENTIFICATION

1. Label all structures on the following figure, and then color all of the bone regions
   different colors.

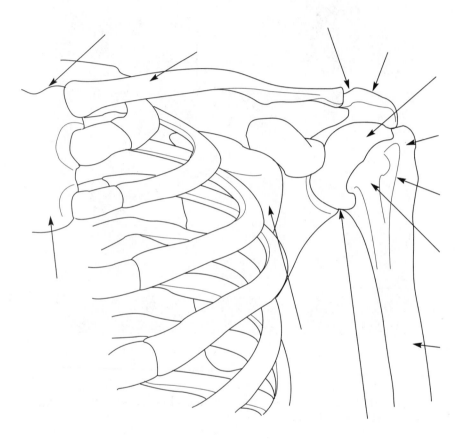

2. Color and label the different regions of the scapula.

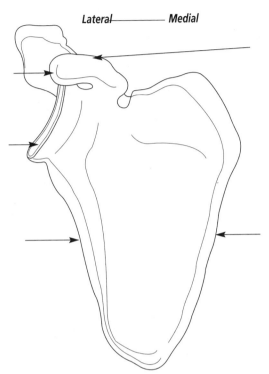

Lateral ———— Medial

A. Right scapula, anterior view

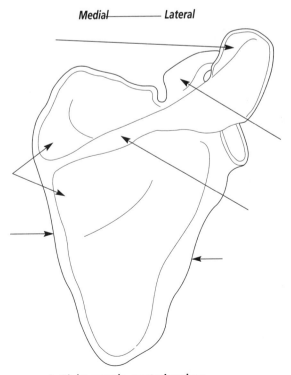

Medial ———— Lateral

B. Right scapula, posterior view

3. Label and color the muscles in the following figures.

Front View   Back View

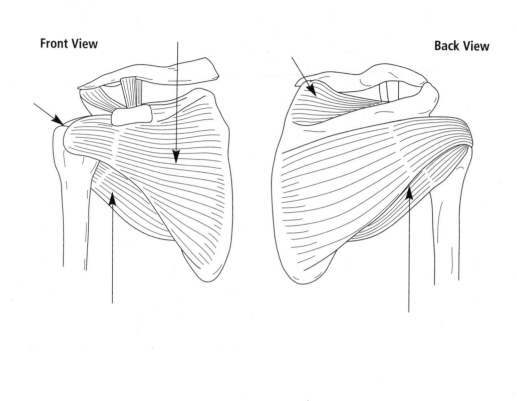

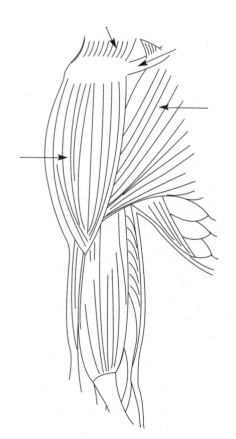
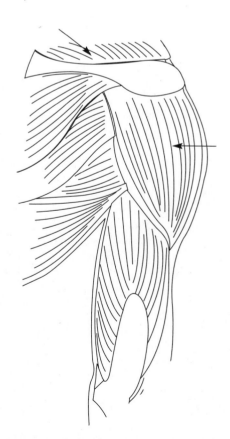

ACTIVITIES

1. Study a model of the shoulder that identifies all the major ligament and tendon attachments. Be able to identify all parts when quizzed.

_____

_____

_____

_____

_____

2. Demonstrate all shoulder movements on yourself and/or another person in the class, identifying the major structures involved in the movement.

_____

_____

_____

_____

_____

ONLINE RESEARCH

■ Choose a disorder involving the shoulder, then go online and find what current research is being done regarding the disorder. Be prepared to report back to the class on any new or alternate treatment methods that are not mentioned in the textbook.

_____

_____

_____

_____

_____

■ Find and print graphics available on the Internet that illustrate the disorders described in the textbook. (Alternative: If you have artistic talent, you may want to illustrate the disorders yourself in ways that differ from what is presented in the text.)

_____

_____

_____

_____

_____

CHAPTER 22

The Chest and Abdomen

KEY CONCEPTS

■ The thoracic cavity contains the lungs and extends from the sternum to the vertebrae of the back. The major organs of the cardiac and respiratory system lie within the thoracic cavity. These vital organs are protected by the bony structures of the ribs. This bony structure also provides support for the torso.

■ The primary function of the respiratory system is to provide for the exchange of oxygen and carbon dioxide in the body. There are many structures that aid in this process.

- The nasal cavity is where air first enters the body. Here the air is warmed, moistened, and filtered.
- Air next passes into the pharynx or throat.
- The larynx or voice box is the next structure through which air passes. It is here that the vocal cords are housed, and as air passes these structures it causes a vibration, creating sound.
- Air then enters the trachea or windpipe. This structure extends down into the chest and branches out into smaller and smaller structures within the lungs.
- The bronchi and bronchioles are these smaller structures. The branching of these structures allows more surface area to be covered.
- At the end of each bronchiole are the alveoli. It is within these structures that the exchange of oxygen and carbon dioxide occurs.
- The lungs are large, cone-shaped organs that hold a tremendous amount of air.
- The pleura is a moist membrane that covers the lungs.
- The mediastinum is the space between the lungs along the median place of the thorax.

■ Respiration is the process by which the body supplies its cells with oxygen and relieves them of carbon dioxide. This takes place through breathing. Breathing is the process by which air enters and leaves the body. Air enters the increased volume within the thoracic cavity upon inhalation or inspiration. During exhalation or expiration, air leaves the body as the volume of the thoracic cavity decreases.

■ Most injuries to the chest are the result of a direct blow and are usually superficial. However, because the chest houses the heart, lungs, and other vital organs, injuries to the chest have the potential to be life-threatening.

(continues)

(continued)

- Chest injuries in athletics are usually the result of a direct blow to the area. These injuries include:
  - Rib contusions, which means bruising of the intercostal muscles between the ribs. The area should be iced for 20 minutes every 3 to 4 hours. The athlete must be closely monitored for signs of a more serious injury or shock.
  - Rib fracture, which is the breakage of one or more ribs. Breaks in three or more consecutive ribs can result in a flail chest. Immediate medical treatment must be sought, as the risk of additional injury is high.
  - Chest contusion, which is bruising of the chest wall. The affected area should be iced for 20 minutes every 3 to 4 hours for 24 to 72 hours. The athlete should be monitored for additional injury and shock.
  - Myocardial contusion, which is bruising of the heart muscle and results from a direct and forceful blow to the middle chest area. It can also result in aortic rupture if the force is great enough to tear or sever the aorta. EMS must be activated.
  - Sudden death syndrome, which is usually the result of an unknown cardiac abnormality. Provide CPR and activate EMS.
  - Pneumothorax, an injury in which air enters the pleural cavity between the chest wall and the lung and causes the lung to collapse. If unrecognized, this can progress to a tension pneumothorax, in which pressure is exerted on the heart and the heart and trachea are pushed away from center. EMS must be activated.
  - Hemothorax, which is similar to a pneumothorax except that blood rather than air enters the pleural space. As with a pneumothorax, EMS must be activated.
  - Pulmonary contusions, which are bruises to the area or structures of the lungs. EMS must be activated.
  - Solar plexus injury (having the wind knocked out), which occurs when a blow to the middle region of the chest affects the nerves in the solar plexus. This condition usually resolves itself in minutes.
  - Hyperventilation, meaning breathing too fast for normal respiratory processes. Treatment should be aimed at calming and relaxing the athlete and encouraging slower breathing.
  - Side stitches, which occur during vigorous exercise and result in pain under the ribs. Treatments vary, and not all treatments work with all athletes. Proper training and conditioning can help prevent side stitches from occurring.
- Abdominal injuries in athletics are rare. However, injuries to the abdomen can affect a number of organs and have the potential to be life-threatening if they go unrecognized. Even mild injuries must be monitored and treated carefully. The solid organs found within the abdominal cavity, when damaged, will bleed profusely and may cause life-threatening hemorrhage.
- Abdominal injuries most often occur during contact sports. These injuries include:
  - Kidney contusion, which is bruising of the kidneys. EMS must be activated.
  - Liver contusion, which is bruising of the liver and is uncommon. This can cause severe bleeding. EMS must be activated.
  - Injuries to the spleen, any of which is a medical emergency. EMS must be activated.
  - Hernia, a protrusion of abdominal tissue through a portion of the abdominal wall. Most hernias eventually require surgery, but a hernia is not normally an emergency.

OUTLINE

I. The Thoracic Cavity

    A. The central area of the thoracic cavity is called the *mediastinum*, which lies between the lungs and extends from the sternum back to the vertebral column.

    B. Each lung is within its own pleural cavity and covered by a thin membrane, the pleura.

II. Ribs and Sternum

    A. Support and protection of the thoracic cavity comes from twelve pairs of ribs, the sternum, and thoracic vertebrae. All ribs are connected posteriorly to the vertebral column.

        1. There are seven pairs of true ribs, directly connected to the sternum anteriorly.

        2. There are five pairs of false ribs, not directly attached to the sternum.

            a. The first three pairs of false ribs are connected to the seventh true rib.

            b. The last two pairs of false ribs have no anterior connection at all and are often referred to as floating ribs.

III. The Respiratory System

    A. The nasal cavity, which is divided in two by the nasal septum, is where air first enters the respiratory system.

        1. Air is filtered by the mucous membrane; dust and dirt particles are swept away by the cilia that line the conchal and nasal cavities.

        2. The air is also moistened by the mucus and warmed by the rich blood supply.

        3. The olfactory nerves at the top of the nasal cavity provide the sense of smell to the brain.

        4. Sinuses branch off the nasal cavity and provide resonance chambers for the sounds made by the vocal cords; they help warm and moisten the inhaled air.

    B. The pharynx, or throat, is the common passageway of air and food. The lower portion of the pharynx houses the epiglottis, a flap of cartilage that closes when swallowing to prevent food from entering the larynx and trachea.

    C. The larynx, or voice box, houses the vocal cords that vibrate as air passes through the opening between them, called the glottis.

    D. The trachea, or windpipe, which is held open by C-shaped cartilage rings, leads air down to the lungs. It is lined with mucus that traps foreign particles, which are swept by cilia back to the pharynx for swallowing.

    E. The bronchi and bronchioles

        1. At the end of the trachea, the tube branches into what are now called bronchus tubes, which continue to subdivide into the smallest tubes of the lungs, called bronchioles.

        2. At the end of each bronchiole are alveolar sacs (alveoli).

    F. The alveoli are air sacs that are found at the ends of the bronchioles. The alveoli are surrounded by a network of blood capillaries, where the exchange of oxygen and carbon dioxide takes place.

    G. The lungs are spongy and porous because of the alveoli and the air they contain. The spongy tissue of the lungs is divided into lobes, three for the right lung and two for the left.

H. The pleura is a thin, moist membrane that covers the lungs. A second pleural membrane lines the inside of the thoracic cavity. Pleurisy is an inflammation of the pleural membranes.

I. The mediastinum is between the lungs and contains the thymus gland, heart, aorta, pulmonary arteries and veins, superior and inferior vena cavae, esophagus, trachea, thoracic duct, lymph nodes, and vessels.

IV. Respiration

A. Respiration refers to the physical and chemical processes that the body uses to provide cells and tissues with oxygen for metabolism and remove the waste carbon dioxide that is produced by metabolic reactions.

B. External respiration involves exchanging gases in the lungs with the outside atmosphere; this process is also called breathing or ventilation.

C. Internal respiration includes the exchange of oxygen and carbon dioxide at the tissues of the body.
   1. Oxygen is used by cells of the body, keeping the oxygen concentration less than that of the incoming blood, so oxygen naturally diffuses from the blood into the cells.
   2. Carbon dioxide is produced by cells of the body, keeping carbon dioxide concentration greater than the incoming blood, so carbon dioxide naturally diffuses from the cells to the blood.

D. Cellular respiration (oxidation) involves the chemical processes of cells using oxygen and producing carbon dioxide.
   1. High energy glucose molecules are dismantled, using oxygen, to their products, carbon dioxide and water.
   2. The water can be used by the body, but the carbon dioxide is the waste product that must be eliminated by the lungs during expiration.

V. Mechanics of Breathing

A. Inhalation/inspiration involves contraction of chest muscles and the diaphragm, which enlarges the thoracic cavity, allowing air to rush in.
   1. The external intercostal muscles lift the ribs upward and outward and the diaphragm contracts, causing it to flatten from its normal dome shape.
   2. This increase in thoracic cavity volume reduces the air pressure within the lungs to less than the atmospheric pressure outside the body.
   3. Because of the pressure difference, air rushes into the lungs.

B. Exhalation (expiration) is a passive process involving no muscle contraction and no expenditure of energy.
   1. The contracted intercostal muscles and diaphragm relax; their elasticity and the elasticity of lung tissue causes the thoracic cavity to get smaller.
   2. The smaller thoracic cavity increases the air pressure within the lungs to greater than the atmospheric pressure outside the body.
   3. Because of the pressure difference, air rushes out of the lungs.

C. Respiratory movements and frequency of respiration
   1. Inspiration and expiration is counted as one respiratory movement.
   2. The normal rate of quiet breathing for an adult is 14 to 20 breaths per minute.
   3. The rate is 40 to 60 for infants and 24 to 26 for 5-year-olds, and can vary as the body's activity and other conditions change.

VI. Control of Breathing

    A. Chemical control depends on the level of carbon dioxide in the blood. The respiratory center of the brain senses the level and increases or decreases the respiratory rate.

    B. There are chemoreceptors on the carotid arteries and aorta that sense blood oxygen levels and can send signals to the respiratory center of the brain.

VII. Lung Capacity and Volume

    A. A spirometer measures the volume and flow of air during inspiration and expiration.

    B. Tidal volume is the amount of air that moves in and out of the lungs with each breath.

    C. Inspiratory reserve volume is the amount of inhaled over and above the tidal volume.

    D. Expiratory reserve volume is the amount of air exhaled over and above the tidal volume.

    E. Vital lung capacity, residual volume, functional residual capacity, and total lung capacity all help to determine if any deficiencies exist.

VIII. Disorders of the Respiratory System

    A. Asthma attacks are the result of a tightening or spasm of the muscles around the airways. The inside lining thickens and gets clogged with thick mucus. It can be controlled with special medications and inhalers, as prescribed by a physician.

    B. Exercise-induced asthma is triggered by vigorous physical activity.

        1. Symptoms include coughing, wheezing, dyspnea (difficulty breathing), and chest tightness.

        2. In athletes, broncoconstriction develops after six to eight minutes of vigorous exercise.

        3. Athletes who have this problem should carry a quick-acting inhaler to relieve symptoms.

IX. Chest (Thorax) Injuries

    A. Rib contusions are caused by a forceful blow to the ribcage that bruises the intercostal muscles.

        1. Symptoms include point tenderness and pain when the chest is palpated and compressed, perhaps with sharp pain during breathing.

        2. Treatment includes ice for 20 minutes every 3 to 4 hours.

        3. It is important to monitor the athlete closely for signs of a more serious injury, including shock.

    B. Rib fractures occur most often from a direct blow to the ribcage.

        1. Fractures of three or more consecutive ribs on the same side of the chest is called flail chest, which does not allow normal inhalation and exhalation of the lungs.

        2. Since displaced fractured ribs can puncture the lung or heart, they must be considered life-threatening.

        3. Symptoms include severe pain during breathing and point tenderness. Crepitus might be felt. Palpation of the ribs with gentle compression will indicate pain at the fracture site.

        4. Treatment involves immediate medical attention. Support the injured site with a pillow and treat for shock until the EMS arrives.

    C. Chest contusions are the most frequent injury to the chest, involving the skin, subcutaneous tissues, muscles, or periosteum of the ribs or sternum.

        1. Symptoms include localized tenderness and possible swelling; there may be no pain during breathing except possibly with very deep breaths. If the contusion is

severe, contusion of the heart muscle must be considered and medical treatment should be sought.

2. Ice should be applied for 15 to 20 minutes every 3 hours for 24 to 72 hours. Compression will keep swelling to a minimum. Monitor for signs of shock.

D. Myocardial contusion and aortic rupture are rare, but possible.

1. Symptoms include severe pain in the chest with rapid onset of shock.
2. Complications can include cardiac tamponade, abnormal heartbeat, congestive heart failure, heart valve damage, heart muscle death, heart wall rupture, and/or weakening of the heart muscle. Aortic rupture is also possible, which normally results in immediate death.
3. Treatment must begin with activating EMS. Be ready to administer CPR if needed.

E. Sudden death syndrome in athletes is usually caused by some form of heart disease such as hypertrophic cardiomyopathy, use of illegal drugs such as cocaine, cerebral aneurysm, and head trauma.

1. Symptoms include chest pain, discomfort during exercise, heart palpitations, shortness of breath, profuse sweating, and loss of consciousness. This condition occurs in individuals who are healthy and show no signs of physical impairment prior to the onset of this condition.
2. Provide CPR until EMS arrives.

F. Pneumothorax occurs when air enters the thoracic cavity between the chest wall and lung, causing the lung to collapse. This is often due to an open chest wound created by a penetrating object or compound rib fracture or by a tear in the lung itself.

1. Three conditions can accompany a chest wound.
   a. A sucking chest wound occurs when air moves through the wound but remains in the pleural space.
   b. A spontaneous pneumothorax is a result of a weakened area of the lung that ruptures.
   c. A tension pneumothorax occurs when air enters the pleural space but cannot exit.
2. Symptoms include severe chest pain, difficulty breathing, cyanosis (bluish skin), unequal expansion of the lungs, and absence of breath sounds on the collapsed side.
3. Activate EMS. Apply an occlusive dressing over any open chest wound. Treat for shock.

G. Hemopneumothorax often accompanies pneumothorax, and refers to blood accumulating in the pleural space. With the loss of blood, the certified athletic trainer must be concerned with the onset of shock.

H. A *pulmonary contusion* is a bruise on the lung caused by a direct blow to the chest, which leads to edema (swelling), hemorrhaging, and increased lung secretions.

1. Symptoms include shortness of breath 24 to 48 hours after the injury, chest pain, coughing, hemoptysis, and rales.
2. Athletes should be transported immediately to the hospital and closely monitored for shock.

I. Blows to the solar (celiac) plexus, or having the wind knocked out, can cause a transitory paralysis of the diaphragm. The condition responds to a few moments of rest and reassurance, without treatment.

J. Hyperventilation is usually brought on by anxiety, stress, or hysteria.

1. The depletion of carbon dioxide from the blood causes chest pain, dizziness, and numbing of the lips, fingers, and toes. The athlete may lose consciousness if it is not controlled.

2. Try to calm the athlete. If he or she loses consciousness, EMS should be contacted. Usually consciousness is regained very quickly.

K. Side stitches can occur during vigorous exercise, especially among novice runners who have not yet established proper pacing and whose breathing tends to be more quick and shallow.

1. Symptoms include pain just under the ribs when running, largely due to a cramping of the diaphragm.

2. Treatment includes stretching, relaxation, altered breathing patterns. What works for one athlete may not work with another.

X. Injury Prevention for the Chest

A. Preventing injury to the chest involves using good, well-maintained, properly fitted equipment.

B. Training in how to protect the chest from injury should be a part of any athlete's overall training routine, especially for contact sports.

XI. The Abdominopelvic Cavity

A. The abdominopelvic cavity is one large cavity bordered superiorly by the diaphragm and inferiorly by the pelvis.

B. Even though there is no physical separation, it is often divided into the abdominal and pelvic cavities.

1. The abdominal cavity includes the stomach, liver, gallbladder, pancreas, spleen, small intestine, appendix, and part of the large intestine.

2. The pelvic cavity includes the urinary bladder, reproductive organs, rectum, and the remainder of the large intestine.

XII. Protection of the Abdominal Organs

A. Usually, the muscular abdominal wall protects organs well enough to avoid injury.

B. Serious injury can occur and may become life-threatening, often affecting organs such as the kidneys, spleen, and liver.

XIII. Organs of the Abdominopelvic Cavity

A. The stomach is located in the upper part of the abdominal cavity just below the left side of the diaphragm.

1. The cardiac sphincter is a circular muscle that opens to let food into the stomach from the esophagus; and at the distal end of the stomach, the pyloric sphincter opens to let food from the stomach into the duodenum.

2. The stomach consists of four layers.

a. The mucous coat lines the inner stomach.

b. The submucosa coat, made of loose areolar connective tissue, is the next layer.

c. The muscular layer actually has three layers of smooth muscle.

d. The serosa is the thick outer layer that protects the stomach from the outside.

B. The small intestine is divided into three segments, the duodenum, the jejunum, and the ileum, and is held in place by the mesentery.

1. The small intestine is the final organ of digestion, leaving the food that is eaten in the form of its basic building blocks such as glucose, amino acids, and fatty acids.

2. These building blocks are small enough for absorption by the walls of the intestines, which are made up of many tiny, fingerlike projections called villi that greatly increase the amount of internal surface area, allowing for the maximum absorption.

C. The pancreas secretes digestive enzymes into the duodenum through the pancreatic duct. It also secretes insulin and glucagon into the blood to regulate blood glucose levels.

D. The liver has many functions.
   1. Its digestive function is to produce bile, which emulsifies fat in the duodenum to help with its digestion. Bile, which contains salts and bilirubin, exits the liver through the hepatic duct and usually moves up the connecting cystic duct for storage in the gallbladder. These ducts join to form the common bile duct.
   2. If this duct is blocked, bile may enter the bloodstream and cause jaundice.
   3. Other liver functions include producing and storing glycogen; detoxifying alcohol, drugs, and other harmful substances; manufacturing blood proteins necessary for blood clotting; preparing urea, a waste product, from amino acid breakdown; and many others.

E. The gallbladder stores and concentrates bile that was produced in the liver. When fat is detected in the duodenum, the gallbladder contracts, releasing its bile into the cystic duct, which ultimately dumps into the duodenum.

F. The large intestine is where undigested and unabsorbed food goes after leaving the ileum.
   1. The first part of the large intestine (colon) is a pouch called the cecum, which connects to the vermiform appendix. The appendix has no digestive function, but it may become inflamed, a condition called appendicitis.
   2. The large intestine (colon) then follows up the right side of the body (ascending colon), across to the left side (transverse colon), then down the left side (descending colon).
   3. The sigmoid colon is an S-shaped portion leading to the rectum, which opens to the anus.

G. The two kidneys are not technically within the abdomen, since they are located behind the peritoneum (retroperitoneal).
   1. Each kidney and the adipose capsule are covered by the renal fascia.
   2. The medial portion of each kidney, concave in shape, is called the hilum, which is where the renal pelvis (a collecting chamber for urine) becomes the ureter (a tube that carries urine to the urinary bladder).
   3. The kidney is divided into the cortex and the medulla.
   4. The nephron (about 1 million per kidney) is the basic structural and functional unit of the kidney; most of the nephron is located within the cortex of the kidney.
      a. Blood in the glomerulus, having come from the afferent arteriole, is pressure filtered, with much of its liquid portion forced into the Bowman's capsule.
      b. The resulting liquid of the Bowman's capsule flows along through the proximal convoluted tubule, the loop of Henle, and the distal convoluted tubule, where most of the useful materials are reabsorbed into the blood that left the glomerulus through the efferent arteriole.

     c. By the time the fluid reaches the collecting tubule, it is in the form of urine and empties ultimately into the renal pelvis, which turns into the ureter.

     d. Two ureters carry urine from the kidneys to the urinary bladder.

  H. The urinary bladder stores urine until it is eliminated from the body through the urethra to the urinary meatus.

  I. Terms referring to regions of the abdominopelvic cavity

    1. The upper epigastric region is just below the sternum.

    2. The umbilical region is located around the navel, or umbilicus.

    3. The hypogastric region, also called the *pubic area*, includes the pelvic cavity.

XIV. Abdominal Injuries

  A. A kidney contusion is the result of a violent blow to the upper posterior abdominal wall.

    1. Symptoms include pain radiating into the lower abdominal region, signs of shock, nausea, vomiting, rigid back muscles, and hematuria.

    2. The athlete must be taken to the hospital immediately.

  B. Liver contusion is a life-threatening injury that needs immediate medical attention.

    1. Symptoms include referred pain just below the right scapula, right shoulder, and substernal area that can radiate to the left side of the chest.

    2. Activate EMS and treat for shock.

  C. Injuries to the spleen are medical emergencies.

    1. Symptoms of spleen injury include pain located in the upper left quadrant. Referred pain may be felt in the left shoulder, radiating one-third of the way down the left arm (Kehr's sign). The athlete may go into shock and have low blood pressure.

    2. Activate EMS for immediate transportation to the hospital. Treat for shock.

  D. A hernia is a protrusion of abdominal tissue through a portion of the abdominal wall.

    1. Inguinal (groin) hernias occur most often in men, femoral hernias most often in women.

    2. Symptoms include a bulge somewhere in the abdomen or pelvic area, or in the scrotum for men. It may cause a sharp or dull pain that worsens when having a bowel movement, during urination, or while lifting heavy objects.

    3. Most hernias require surgery, and though it is not an emergency it can become serious if not treated.

VOCABULARY REVIEW

Matching

Match the terms on the right with the definitions on the left. Terms may be used once, more than once, or not at all.

_____ 1. The passage that brings bile to the duodenum

_____ 2. The tubular structure that ascends to the cortex from the loop of Henle

_____ 3. The partition between the two nasal cavities

_____ 4. Nerve that suppies the nasal mucosa and provides a sense of smell

_____ 5. The area of the body that contains the stomach, liver, gallbladder, pancreas, spleen, small intestine, appendix, and part of the large intestine

_____ 6. The use of oxygen to release energy from the cell

_____ 7. The opposite of what is expected

_____ 8. The double-walled capsule around the glomerulus of a nephron

_____ 9. A cluster of nerves located in the upper middle region of the abdomen; also known as the solar plexus

_____ 10. The structure that carries blood from the glomerulus

_____ 11. Bruising over the central area of the chest as a result of a compressive blow to the chest

_____ 12. The upper region of the abdomen

_____ 13. The structure in the nephron that collects urine from the distal convoluted tubule

_____ 14. Breathing; the act of inspiration and expiration

_____ 15. The space within the vocal cords of the larynx

_____ 16. The accumulation of blood in the pleural space

_____ 17. The area from below the diaphragm to the pubic floor, with no separation between the abdomen and pelvis

_____ 18. The indentation along the medial border of the kidney

A. abdominal cavity

B. abdominopelvic cavity

C. afferent arteriole

D. bilirubin

E. Bowman's capsule

F. bronchoconstriction

G. cardiac sphincter

H. cardiac tamponade

I. celiac plexus

J. cellular respiration

K. chest contusion

L. cecum

M. collecting tubule

N. common bile duct

O. distal convoluted tubule

P. efferent arteriole

Q. epigastric region

R. exercise-induced asthma

S. external respiration

T. false ribs

U. flail chest

V. glomerulus

W. glottis

X. hemopneumothorax

Y. hilum

Z. hypertrophic cardiomyopathy

AA. hyperventilation

BB. hypogastric region

CC. internal respiration

DD. Kehr's sign

EE. kidney contusion

_____ 19. Located behind the peritoneum

_____ 20. Structure that takes blood from the renal artery to the Bowman's capsule

_____ 21. One of two pigments that determines the color of bile; reddish in color

_____ 22. Thickening of the cardiac muscle

_____ 23. Narrowing of the bronchioles

_____ 24. Circular muscle fibers around the cardiac end of the esophagus

_____ 25. The buildup of fluid in the pericardium

_____ 26. Breathing at a faster rate than is required for proper exchange of oxygen and carbon dioxide

_____ 27. The amount of air that moves in and out of the lungs with each breath

_____ 28. The portion of the colon that veers left across the abdomen to the spleen

_____ 29. The lower region of the abdomen

_____ 30. Bruising the kidney

_____ 31. The proximal convoluted tubule that descends into the medulla

_____ 32. The intrapleural space separating the sternum in front and the vertebral column behind

_____ 33. A fracture of three or more consecutive ribs on the same side of the chest

_____ 34. A collection of porous capillaries within the Bowman's capsule of a nephron

_____ 35. Bruising of the heart muscle

_____ 36. The area of the body containing the urinary bladder, reproductive organs, rectum, and the remainder of the large intestine

_____ 37. Airway narrowing as a result of increased physical activity

_____ 38. A pouch at the proximal end of the large intestine

_____ 39. The space between the lung and chest wall

_____ 40. Inflammation of the lining of the lungs

_____ 41. A wormlike sac that opens into the cecum

FF. loop of Henle

GG. mediastinum

HH. myocardial contusion

II. nasal septum

JJ. olfactory nerves

KK. oxidation

LL. paradoxical

MM. pelvic cavity

NN. pleural space

OO. pleurisy

PP. pneumothorax

QQ. proximal convoluted tubule

RR. pyloric sphincter

SS. renal fascia

TT. renal pelvis

UU. respiration

VV. retroperitoneal

WW. rib contusion

XX. rib fracture

YY. side stitches

ZZ. sigmoid colon

AAA. spirometer

BBB. spleen

CCC. spontaneous pneumothorax

DDD. sucking chest wound

EEE. sudden death syndrome

FFF. tension pneumothorax

GGG. tidal volume

HHH. transverse colon

III. true ribs

JJJ. umbilical area

KKK. urinary bladder

LLL. urinary meatus

MMM. vermiform appendix

_____ 42. The rapid collapse and death of an otherwise healthy person; usually the result of an unknown congenital disorder

_____ 43. Air that enters the pleural space between the chest wall and lung

_____ 44. The twisted, tubular branch off the Bowman's capsule

_____ 45. The funnel-shaped structure at the beginning of the ureter

_____ 46. The physical and chemical process by which the body supplies its cells and tissues with oxygen and relieves them of carbon dioxide

_____ 47. The exchange of carbon dioxide and oxygen between the cells and the lymph surrounding them; the oxidative process of energy in the cells

_____ 48. Pain that radiates to the left shoulder and two-thirds of the way down the left arm, resulting from a kidney contusion

_____ 49. A break in the bony structure of the thorax

_____ 50. Pain that occurs just under the ribcage during vigorous exercise

_____ 51. The S-shaped portion of the colon

_____ 52. A valve that regulates the entrance of food from the stomach to the duodenum

_____ 53. The tough, fibrous tissue covering the kidney

_____ 54. A device that measures the volume and flow of air during inspiration and expiration

_____ 55. The rupture of a weakened area of the lung, which allows air to escape into the pleural space

_____ 56. An open wound in the chest that allows air to enter and become trapped in the pleural space

_____ 57. The opening to the urethra

_____ 58. The entrapment of air in the pleural space, causing pressure on the lung and heart

_____ 59. The area located around the navel

_____ 60. A muscular, membrane-lined sac used to hold urine

Crossword Puzzle

Identify the terms described in the puzzle clues, then write the letters in the boxes. (Many terms are more than one word.)

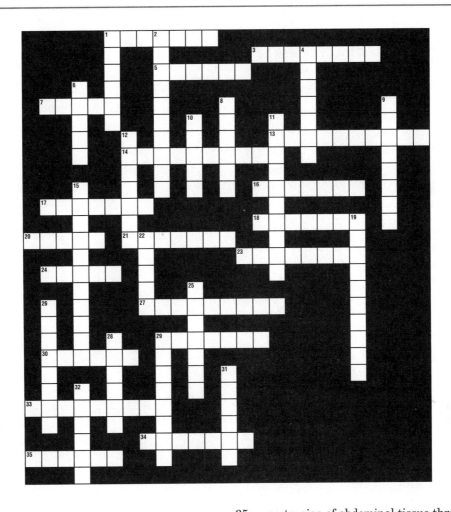

Across

1. air sacs _____
3. yellowish color _____
5. lung membrane _____
7. last portion of the small intestine
   _____
13. the smallest subdivision of the bronchus
    _____
14. prevents food from entering the larynx
    _____
16. the tube from the bladder to outside the body
    _____
17. throat _____
18. the esophagus dumps food into this organ
    _____
20. hairlike projections within the small intestine
    _____
21. inner portion of an organ _____
23. first part of the small intestine _____
24. a crackling sound during breathing _____
27. portion of colon on the right side of the body
    _____
29. windpipe _____
30. outer portion of an organ _____
33. blood in the urine _____
34. cavities filled with air around the nasal cavity
    _____

35. a protrusion of abdominal tissue through the
    abdominal wall _____

Down

1. airway obstruction due to an inflammatory
   reaction _____
2. exhalation _____
4. structural and functional unit of the kidney
   _____
6. a pouch at the beginning of the large intestine
   _____
8. the duct to the gallbladder _____
9. primary branch of the trachea _____
10. large intestine _____
11. the passage of a substance into body fluids
    and tissues _____
12. the second section of small intestine _____
15. stores bile _____
19. coughing up blood _____
22. swelling _____
25. the duct leading from the liver carrying bile
    _____
26. a polysaccharide stored in the liver _____
28. the part of the colon that opens to the anus
    _____
29. another name for chest _____
31. the tube from kidney to bladder _____
32. voice box _____

ANATOMY IDENTIFICATION

1. Label and color all structures of the ribs and sternum.

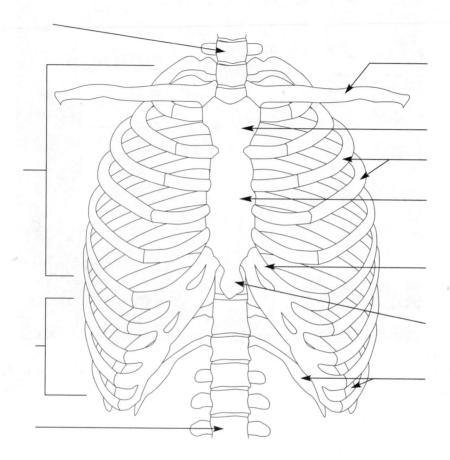

2. Label and color all respiratory organs and structures.

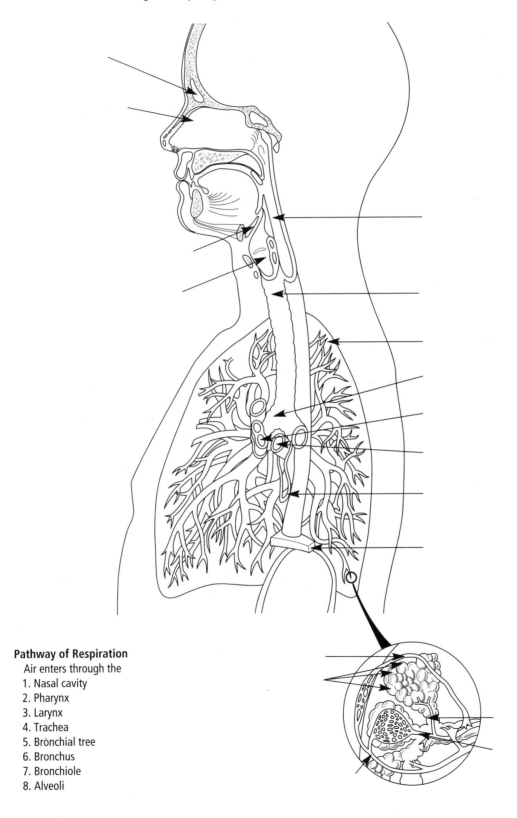

Pathway of Respiration
Air enters through the
1. Nasal cavity
2. Pharynx
3. Larynx
4. Trachea
5. Bronchial tree
6. Bronchus
7. Bronchiole
8. Alveoli

3. For the following figure, label and color all parts of the digestive system.

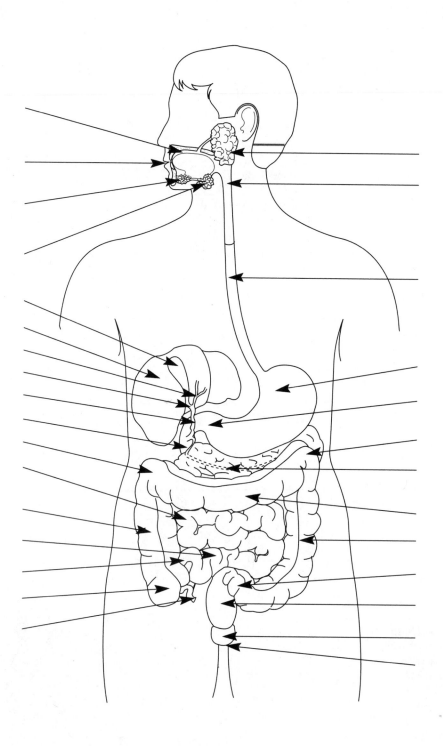

ACTIVITIES

1. Using the model of a skeleton, become familiar with all of the bones mentioned in the textbook, their relationships to each other, and the joints they make. Be able to demonstrate your knowledge without the use of notes, diagrams, or other outside material.

_____

_____

_____

_____

_____

2. The internal organs of mammals are nearly identically arranged to those in the human body. Dissect or watch the dissection of a fetal pig or rat. Find as many of the thoracic and abdominal structures mentioned in the textbook as possible, and be able to identify them.

_____

_____

_____

_____

_____

ONLINE RESEARCH

■ Research current or alternative treatments of thoracic and abdominal injuries. Note any differences from what is described in the textbook.

_____

_____

_____

_____

CHAPTER 23

The Head and Face

KEY CONCEPTS

- The head can be divided into two anatomical groups: the face and the cranium. The face includes the structures of the eye, nose, mouth, ears, and jaw. The cranium includes the brain, skull, and spinal cord attachments.

- Eye injuries:
  - Dirt and debris can become imbedded into the structures of the eye and cause pain or a corneal abrasion. A corneal abrasion is a cut or scratch on the cornea. Attempts can be made to wash objects out of the eye by splashing water into the eye. However, imbedded objects should not be removed and the athlete should be instructed to see a physician.
  - A blow or contusion to the eye often results in a black eye. Application of a cold compress for 15 minutes immediately after the injury will aid in reducing pain and swelling.
  - Cuts, punctures, or abrasions to the eye or eyelid can cause infection and blindness. These are medical emergencies and the athlete should be promptly transported to a medical facility.
  - An orbital blow-out fracture is a break in the bones that house the eye. Immediate treatment consists of bandaging both eyes and applying an ice compress for 15 to 20 minutes. The athlete should seek immediate treatment from an ophthalmologist.
  - Hyphemia is the buildup of blood in the anterior chamber of the eye. Treatment will depend on the cause, but the athlete should seek the care of an ophthalmologist.
  - Conjunctivitis is an infection of the outermost layer of the eye. This is usually contagious and requires medical attention.

- Ear injuries:
  - Cauliflower ear is a deformity caused by damage to the cartilage in the outer ear. Drainage of blood buildup will help keep this from occurring if done early.
  - Swimmer's ear is an infection of the skin covering the outer ear canal. The ear must be kept dry, as moisture will irritate and prolong the problem.
  - Foreign bodies may become lodged in the ear. Treatment is removal of the object, but the method of removal will depend on the type of material lodged in the ear and how far in the ear it is lodged.
  - Tympanic rupture is perforation of the tympanic membrane. The athlete should immediately be taken to a physician for treatment.

(continues)

(continued)

- Nasal injuries:
  - Epistaxis (nosebleed) is a concern only when the bleeding is difficult to stop or is recurrent. Infection control procedures must be maintained when dealing with a nosebleed. The athlete should sit down, lean forward, and squeeze the soft portion of the nose to stop the bleeding.
  - A nasal fracture is a break in the bone or damage to the cartilaginous structures of the nose. Control bleeding, apply ice, and refer the athlete to a physician for further treatment.
- Injuries to the mouth and jaw:
  - A jaw fracture is a break in the lower jaw bone. The athlete should be immobilized, ice should be applied, and the athlete should be monitored for shock. Treatment by a physician is necessary.
  - Dislocation of the temporomandibular joint can cause severe pain, swelling, and deformity. Apply ice and refer the athlete to a physician for treatment.
  - Injuries to the teeth can result in loose, chipped, or missing teeth. If a tooth is knocked out or hanging from the socket, place the tooth back in the socket, maintaining pressure to keep it in place. If that is not possible, wrap the tooth in moist gauze so the athlete can take it to the dentist for possible reimplantation.
- Signs of concussion include: unawareness of surroundings, date, time, or place; loss of consciousness; confusion; amnesia; headache; dizziness; nausea; unsteadiness/loss of balance; ringing in the ears; double vision or seeing flashes of light; sleepiness; sleep disturbance; convulsions; exhibition of inappropriate emotions; vacant stare; and slurred speech.

OUTLINE

I. The Head and Face

   A. The term *head injury* may be used to describe damage to the scalp, skull, or brain, usually as the result of the application of a sudden force to the head.

   B. The head can be divided into two anatomical groups: the face and the cranium.

     1. The face includes the eyes, ears, nose, jaw, and mouth.

     2. The cranium includes the brain and spinal cord attachments.

II. The Eye

   A. The eye is protected in many ways from the outside world.

     1. Eyebrows, eyelashes, and eyelids provide physical barriers to objects that might get into the eye.

     2. Tears, produced by nearby lacrimal glands, keep the eye moist, wash away small foreign objects that make it into the eye, and contain an enzyme capable of destroying bacteria.

     3. Glands along the border of each eyelid secrete a substance that helps smooth the surface and lubricate the eye. An infection of these glands is called a sty.

    4. The conjunctiva is a thin membrane that covers the entire front of the eye and part of the inner eyelid.

B. The sclera, or white of the eye, is a thick, fibrous layer that maintains the shape of the eye and protects the structures within. It is attached to the extrinsic eye muscles that are responsible for the eye movements.

C. The cornea is continuous with the sclera, but is transparent, allowing light to pass through into the inner structures of the eye. Its convex shape works along with the lens to create a sharp image on the retina of the eye.

D. The choroid coat lines the inner sclera and is darkly pigmented to prevent random reflections of light entering the eye's inner structures.

    1. The choroid coat is continuous with the iris—a variably pigmented layer that has a central opening, called the pupil—through which light passes to get to the eye's internal structures.

    2. The intrinsic eye muscles are located within the iris, allowing it to change the size of the pupil and responded to the amount of light available.

E. The lens is a transparent, crystalline structure attached by suspensory ligaments to the ciliary body that controls the thickness of the lens.

    1. As the lens increases in thickness, the eye is able to sharply focus nearby objects onto the retina.

    2. The anterior chamber and the posterior chamber are filled with a watery fluid called the aqueous humor.

    3. Behind the lens is an area filled with a jellylike substance, called the vitreous humor, that extends back to the retina and helps maintain the shape of the eye.

F. The retina is the thin layer of cells located between the vitreous humor and the choroid coat that contains the light-sensitive cells called rods and cones.

    1. The rods are sensitive to dim light; since there is only one type of rod, they cannot distinguish colors.

    2. The cones are active in bright light. There are three different kinds of cones, each sensitive to a different range of light frequencies, that allow for color vision.

    3. The fovea centralis is an area of the retina especially rich in cones, where the retina is the thinnest, providing the sharpest vision. The other parts of the retina provide our peripheral vision, which is not as sharp.

    4. The optic disc is located where the nerve fibers from the rods and cones leave the eye and enter the optic nerve. The optic disc has no rods or cones, so it is also called the blind spot.

III. Pathway of Vision

IV. Eye Injuries

A. Specks in the eyes can cause corneal abrasions, scratches, or cuts on the cornea.

    1. Objects should be washed out by splashing clean water into the eye.

    2. If the object cannot be removed, or is imbedded in the eye, the athlete should see a doctor immediately.

B. Blows (contusions) to the eye are common in sports. The eye is located in a deep socket call the orbit.

    1. Symptoms include pain, swelling, and discoloration.

    2. Treatment includes applying a cold compress immediately for 15 minutes, and again each hour as needed. If there is discoloration or blackening of the eye, the athlete should consult a physician immediately.

C. Cuts, punctures, and abrasions of the eye or eyelid are medical emergencies and require prompt transport to the nearest medical facility.

D. An orbital blow-out fracture consists of a fracture of the bones of the eye socket and is usually secondary to a blunt blow from a relatively large object.

    1. Symptoms include pain, tenderness, swelling, bruising, double vision (diplopia), protrusion of the eye (proptosis), and/or numbness in the cheek and upper jaw areas.

    2. Bandage both eyes and apply an ice compress for 15 to 20 minutes. The athlete should be sent to an ophthalmologist.

E. Hyphema refers to bleeding in the anterior chamber of the eye, due to bleeding of the vessels of the iris.

    1. Symptoms include the athlete complaining of dramatically decreased vision.

    2. Athletes with hyphema should be seen by an ophthalmologist, even though the blood is often reabsorbed over a period of days to weeks.

F. Conjunctivitis, or pinkeye, is an infection of the conjunctiva, which can be caused by a virus, bacteria, or an allergic reaction.

    1. The viral and bacterial forms are typically contagious.

    2. Symptoms include eye discomfort followed by redness and inflammation of the conjunctiva. After a day or so, a white, yellow, or green discharge from the eyes may be present.

    3. Treatment requires medical attention and depends on the cause.

V. The Ear

A. The ear consists of three parts: the outer ear, the middle ear, and the inner ear.

B. The outer ear is composed of the pinna and the ear canal.

    1. The pinna (auricle) is the visible part of the ear composed of folds of skin and cartilage.

    2. The ear canal (also called the meatus) is a short tube leading to the tympanic membrane (eardrum). It produces wax that, along with tiny hairs in the canal, help trap dust and small foreign bodies.

C. The middle ear is an air-filled space between the eardrum and the inner ear. Its hearing structures consist of three small bones called ossicles. It contains the eardrum, hammer, anvil, stirrup, and eustachian tube.

    1. The malleus (hammer) is attached to the inside of the eardrum.

    2. The incus (anvil) connects the malleus to the stapes.

    3. The stapes (stirrup) is the third bone, which attaches the incus to the oval window of the inner ear.

    4. The eustachian tube connects the middle ear to the throat. It is closed unless the person is swallowing or yawning. It then opens the space of the middle ear to outside air, equalizing air pressure in the middle ear to that of the outside.

D. The inner ear consists of an extremely intricate series of structures contained within the bones of the skull.

    1. The cochlea is a coiled tube containing the sensory nerves for the sense of hearing.

    2. The semicircular canals contain the sensory nerves for detecting how the head is moving.

      3. A cavity known as the vestibule contains the sensory nerves that inform the brain about the current position of the head.

      4. These structures are connected to the vestibulocochlear nerve, which carries the sensory information to the nearby brain.

VI. Injuries to the Ear

  A. Cauliflower ear is caused by the destruction of the underlying cartilage of the outer ear (pinna). Blood collects between the cartilage and skin, causing a thickening of the entire outer ear.

      1. Symptoms include a blood clot under the skin of the ear, which will eventually cause the ear cartilage to die and shrivel up, since the skin is its only blood supply.

      2. Treatment of the hematoma (blood clot) is to drain it through an incision in the ear and apply a compressive dressing to sandwich the two sides of skin against the cartilage.

  B. Swimmer's ear is an infection of the skin covering the outer ear canal. The ear needs to be kept dry, since moisture will irritate and prolong the problem.

  C. Foreign bodies in the ear, including insects, can be difficult to remove because of the small size of the ear canal.

      1. Symptoms include mild to severe ear pain, drainage from the ear, fever, nausea and vomiting, coughing, tearing from the eye, dizziness, and a foul odor from the ear caused by infection.

      2. Treatment involves anything from gentle flushing of the ear canal with warm water to surgery to remove the object.

  D. Tympanic rupture is most often caused by a middle ear infection, but may be due to trauma.

      1. Symptoms include severe ear pain and sudden drainage, if caused by an infection.

      2. Treatment, whatever the cause, involves immediate transport to a physician for evaluation and treatment.

VII. The Nose

  A. The outer nose is composed of bone, cartilage, and skin, and projects from the front of the face, making it susceptible to injury.

  B. The human nose serves as an air passage for the respiratory system and provides the brain with the sense of smell.

VIII. Injuries to the Nose

  A. Epistaxis is the medical term for nosebleed, though it usually refers to recurrent nosebleeds or those difficult to stop.

      1. A sign of posterior epistaxis is an athlete complaining of swallowing blood. There is no way for the certified athletic trainer to stop this type of nosebleed. Posterior nosebleeds can be life-threatening and should be considered a medical emergency.

      2. For anterior epistaxis, the athlete should sit and lean slightly forward. The athlete should squeeze the soft portion of the nose for about 5 minutes and repeat if necessary. A cold compress across the bridge of the nose can help.

  B. Nasal fractures and septal deviations occur as the result of direct blows or as the result of falls. The nasal bones are the most commonly fractured bony structures of the face.

1. Symptoms include signs of deformity, swelling, skin laceration, ecchymosis, epistaxis, and leakage of cerebrospinal fluid (CSF).

2. Treatment begins with careful, direct pressure, the application of ice, and getting the athlete to sit with the head tilted slightly forward. The athlete should be sent to a physician for additional care and treatment.

IX. The Mouth and Jaw

A. The mouth includes structures like the soft and hard palate, mucous membranes, tongue, teeth, lips, and cheeks.

B. The upper jaw includes the maxilla bone, which is fixed to the skull.

C. The lower jaw is the mandible bone, which is attached at a moveable joint on the temporal bone of the skull, called the temporomandibular joint (TMJ).

X. Injuries to the Mouth and Jaw

A. Jaw fractures usually include two fractures, one direct, and one indirect. The indirect fracture is usually located near one of the condyles of the mandible close to the joint.

1. Symptoms include severe pain, swelling, blood at the base of the teeth near the fracture, deformity, tenderness, and sometimes numbness.

2. Treatment includes immobilization, application of ice, and treatment for shock. The athlete should be transported to a physician immediately.

B. Temporomandibular joint injuries change the function of most mouth parts, since they all work together to open and close the mouth.

1. Symptoms include malocclusion (the teeth not coming together), muscle imbalance, postural imbalance, severe pain, deformity, swelling, a feeling of popping, and difficulty opening and closing the mouth.

2. Treatment includes application of ice and referral to a physician.

C. Injuries to the teeth are greatly reduced by the use of mouth guards. However, when mouth guards are not required, they are often not worn.

1. Symptoms include loose, chipped, or missing teeth and pain.

2. Treatment includes putting the tooth back into the socket if it is knocked out or hanging from the socket, and transport immediately to a dentist. Otherwise, the tooth should be wrapped in a sterile, moist gauze and the athlete should take it to the dentist. The longer the tooth is out of the mouth, the less likely it is that the tooth can be saved.

XI. The Head

A. The cranium is a collection of bones fused together to protect the brain.

1. The frontal bone makes up the forehead, and the temporal bone forms the sides and base of the skull.

2. The mastoid sinuses are the air-filled spaces within the mastoid process of the temporal bone.

3. The spinal cord passes through the occipital bone through the foramen magnum.

4. The parietal bone is the largest bone in the skull.

5. All cranial bones are joined at immovable joints called sutures.

B. The brain is subdivided into portions, each having its own function.

1. The brain stem is the most basic part of the human brain and controls many of the life-sustaining functions of the body, such as breathing and heartbeat.

2. The cerebellum controls muscular coordination.

3. The cerebrum is divided into a left and right hemisphere and is the center for all complex brain activities and sensory reception.

4. The meninges are three membranes that surround the brain and spinal cord. The pia mater, arachnoid, and dura mater are layers that pad the brain for protection.

XII. Head Injuries

A. Scalp injuries may or may not involve the skull or brain. Common athletic injuries to the scalp are contusions and lacerations.

1. Symptoms include local tenderness, swelling, and bleeding between the skin and underlying tissue.

2. Treatment includes locating the source of the bleeding, and controlling it by using direct pressure. Care should be taken not to depress the fracture site with added pressure.

B. Skull fractures range from a simple linear fracture to a severe compound depressed fracture, with bone fragments lacerating brain tissue.

1. Symptoms include bleeding or cerebrospinal fluid drainage from the ear or nose.

2. Treatment includes activating EMS and treating for shock.

XIII. Brain Injuries

A. Injuries include cerebral concussions and cerebral contusions, which can result in a contrecoup.

B. Concussions occur commonly in sport activities.

1. Symptoms can include being unaware of surroundings, date, time, or place; loss of consciousness; confusion; amnesia; headache; dizziness; nausea; unsteadiness/ loss of balance; ringing in the ears; double vision or seeing flashes of light; sleepiness; sleep disturbance; convulsions; exhibiting inappropriate emotions; vacant stare; slurred speech.

2. Several different scales exist for grading concussions:

a. The Glasgow Coma Scale (GCS) evaluates eye opening, motor responses, and verbal responses.

b. The American College of Surgeons Committee on Trauma has adopted the AVPU method which investigates whether the individual is alert, responsive to verbal stimuli, responsive to painful stimuli, or unresponsive.

3. Treatment includes reviewing the history of the injury, inspection, palpation of cervical vertebrae and musculature, and neurological screening of sensory and motor function and pupil size. Raised intracranial pressure and temporal lobe herniation will cause compression of the oculomotor nerve, resulting in pupillary dilation.

4. Treatment includes removal from the game or practice, monitoring for deterioration, medical evaluation, and using a medically supervised, stepwise process to determine return to play status.

5. Amnesia may take the form of retrograde amnesia, in which there is a loss of memory for events that occurred before the injury; or antegrade amnesia, in which there is a loss of memory for events occurring immediately after awakening from a loss of consciousness.

6. Postconcussion syndrome may develop following a concussion, and the athlete should be monitored for symptoms periodically.

C. Brain contusions, or bruising of the brain, may result in lack of nerve function of the bruised portion, but usually will not result in a loss of consciousness. Symptoms include numbness, weakness, loss of memory, aphasia (loss of speech or comprehension), or general misbehavior.

D. Hemorrhage (bleeding) is potentially life-threatening.

1. A subdural hematoma develops when bridging cerebral vessels that travel from the brain to the dura mater are torn. It is the most frequent cause of death from trauma in athletics.

2. An epidural hematoma develops when a dural artery is ruptured; it is often associated with a skull fracture.

3. An intracranial hematoma develops when blood vessels within the brain are damaged.

4. All hematomas can cause an increase in intracranial pressure that can lead to death or disability if not dealt with appropriately.

E. Secondary impact syndrome (SIS) involves rapid swelling and herniation of the brain after a second head injury occurs before the symptoms of a previous injury have been resolved.

1. The second injury may not even be a blow directly to the head, but rather to a nearby area, such as the chest or back, that causes the head to react to the blow.

2. Prevention is the only sure cure. Athletes must not be allowed to participate in contact or collision activities until all cerebral symptoms have subsided.

VOCABULARY REVIEW

Matching 1

Match the terms on the right with the definitions on the left. Terms may be used once, more than once, or not at all.

_____ 1. Bruising or laceration of the brain tissues caused by impact from the skull on underlying tissue

_____ 2. The most basic part of the human brain

_____ 3. Deformity of the ear caused by destruction of the underlying cartilage of the outer ear

_____ 4. The muscles responsible for moving the eye within the orbital socket

_____ 5. Injury to the brain from a forceful impact, causing temporary dysfunction

_____ 6. A substance that is found in the ventricles of the brain, which acts as a shock absorber for the brain and spinal cord

_____ 7. The middle layer of the eye

A. antegrade amnesia
B. anterior chamber
C. brain stem
D. cauliflower ear
E. cerebral concussion
F. cerebral contusion
G. cerebrospinal fluid (CSF)
H. choroid coat
I. ciliary body
J. ear canal
K. extrinsic eye muscles
L. foramen magnum
M. frontal bone

_____ 8. An area of the eye devoid of visual reception; also known as the blind spot

_____ 9. A condition following a concussion exhibited by a persistent headache, dizziness, fatigue, irritability, and impaired memory or lack of concentration

_____ 10. A structure that surrounds the lens of the eye and contains muscles that control the shape of the lens

_____ 11. The passageway for sound in the ear

_____ 12. Large opening at the base of the skull through which the spinal cord passes

_____ 13. A loss of memory of the events that occurred immediately after the injury

_____ 14. Damage to blood vessels within the brain

_____ 15. Perforation of the tympanic membrane (eardrum) between the middle ear and the ear canal

_____ 16. The space between the cornea and iris

_____ 17. The strong anterior bone in the skull that makes up the forehead

_____ 18. The front portion of the roof of the mouth

_____ 19. An extremely intricate series of structures contained deep within the bones of the skull; consists of the cochlea, semicircular canals, and other organs of balance

_____ 20. A transparent, gelatin-like substance that fills the greater part of the eyeball

_____ 21. The back portion of the roof of the mouth

_____ 22. The muscles that help the iris control the amount of light entering the pupil

_____ 23. An air-filled space within the mastoid process of the temporal bone behind the ears

N. Glasgow Coma Scale (GCS)

O. hard palate

P. inner ear

Q. intracranial hematoma

R. intracranial hemorrhaging

S. intrinsic eye muscles

T. loss of consciousness (LOC)

U. mastoid sinus

V. optic disc

W. postconcussion syndrome

X. soft palate

Y. tympanic rupture

Z. vitreous humor

Matching 2

Match the terms on the right with the definitions on the left. Terms may be used once, more than once, or not at all.

_____ 1. An opening; in this instance, the opening to the ear canal

_____ 2. The watery fluid found in the anterior and posterior chambers of the eye

_____ 3. A maze of winding passageways that can be found in the ear

_____ 4. An area of the eye devoid of visual reception; also known as the optic disc

_____ 5. The area of the retina that provides the sharpest vision and consists mostly of cones

_____ 6. A small cavity between the eardrum and inner ear containing the hammer, anvil, and stirrup

_____ 7. Widening of the pupils caused by increased intracranial pressure compressing the third cranial nerve

_____ 8. The most posterior bone in the skull

_____ 9. The space between the iris and the lens

_____ 10. A loss of memory of events that occurred before the injury

_____ 11. Rapid swelling and herniation of the brain after a second head injury occurs before the first injury has resolved

_____ 12. A mechanism of injury in which the brain rebounds off the other side of the skull from the initial impact

_____ 13. Structures in the inner ear involved with equilibrium

_____ 14. A collection of blood between the surface of the brain and dura mater

_____ 15. The passageway from the throat to the middle ear, which equalizes the pressure in the middle ear

_____ 16. The structures that hold the lens of the eye in place

_____ 17. The visible part of the ear; consists of the pinna (auricle)

A. aqueous humor

B. blind spot

C. contrecoup

D. corneal abrasion

E. dura mater

F. epidural hematoma

G. eustachian tube

H. fovea centralis

I. labyrinth

J. meatus

K. middle ear

L. occipital bone

M. outer ear

N. posterior chamber

O. pupillary dilation

P. retrograde amnesia

Q. secondary impact syndrome (SIS)

R. semicircular canal

S. subdural hematoma

T. suspensory ligaments

U. sutures

V. swimmer's ear

W. temporal bone

X. temporomandibular joint (TMJ)

Y. tinnitus

Z. tympanic membrane

AA. vestibule

BB. vestibulocochlear nerve

_____ 18. Immovable joints, composed of connective tissue, in the skull where the cranial bones meet

_____ 19. An infection of the skin covering the outer ear canal

_____ 20. The cranial bone that forms part of the base of the skull behind and at the sides of the face

_____ 21. The area where the mandible connects with the temporal bone of the skull

_____ 22. The outermost membrane covering the spinal cord and brain

_____ 23. The membrane that separates the external ear from the middle ear; also known as the eardrum

_____ 24. A collection of blood between the skull and dura mater

_____ 25. A small cavity of the inner ear that contains some of the organs of balance

Crossword Puzzle

Identify the terms described in the puzzle clues, then write the letters in the boxes. (Many terms are more than one word.)

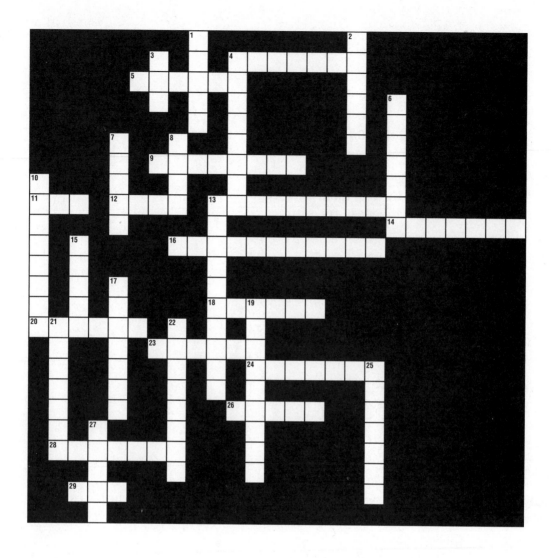

Across

4. upper jaw bone _____
5. helps the lens focus light _____
9. largest portion of the human brain _____
11. infection of a gland along the eyelid
    _____
12. changes the size of the pupil _____
13. part of the brain that coordinates
    muscle movement _____
14. loss of speech or comprehension
    _____
16. outermost layer of the eye _____
18. stirrup _____
20. hammer _____
23. contains rods and cones _____
24. the bony skull _____
26. anvil _____
28. the visible part of the ear _____
29. inner layer of the meninges _____

Down

1. cells responsible for color vision _____
2. the bone that attaches to the eardrum
   _____
3. a cell sensitive to dim light _____
4. lower jaw bone _____
6. buildup of blood in the eye's anterior chamber
   _____
7. the middle bone of the middle ear _____
8. attached to suspensory ligaments _____
10. small bones _____
13. a mild traumatic brain injury _____
15. opening in the iris _____
17. tympanic membrane _____
19. middle layer of the meninges _____
21. spiral organ that houses the sensory nerves
    for hearing _____
22. three membranes that protect the brain
23. the white of the eye _____
27. a deep socket that houses the eye
    _____

ANATOMY IDENTIFICATION

1. Label and color the structures of the eye.

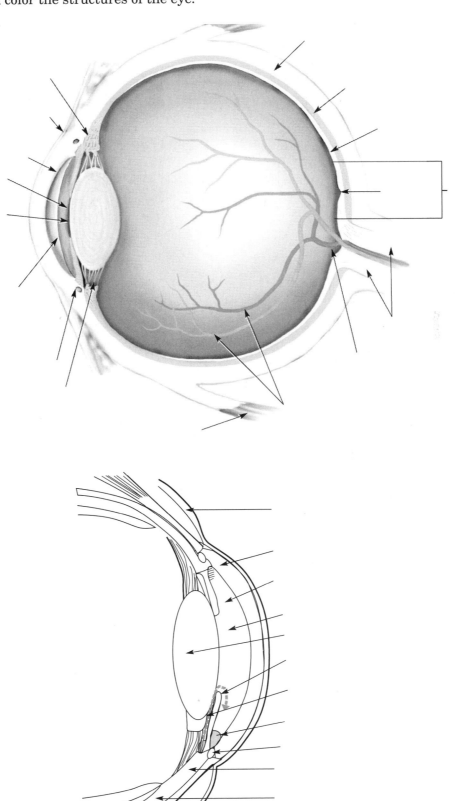

2. Label and color the individual bones of the skull and jaw.

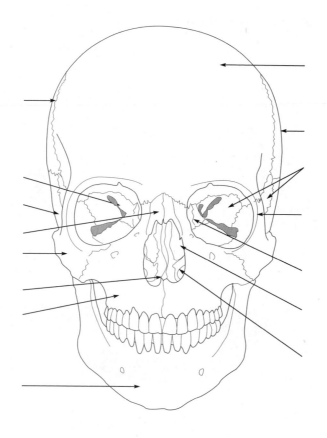

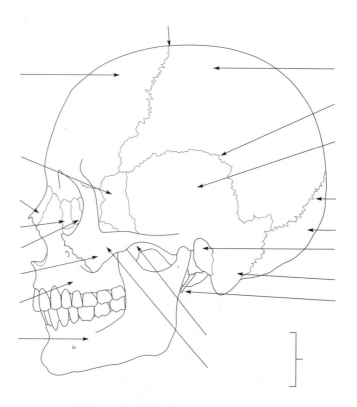

3. Label and color the structures of the ear. Use brackets to indicate the location of the external ear, middle ear, and inner ear.

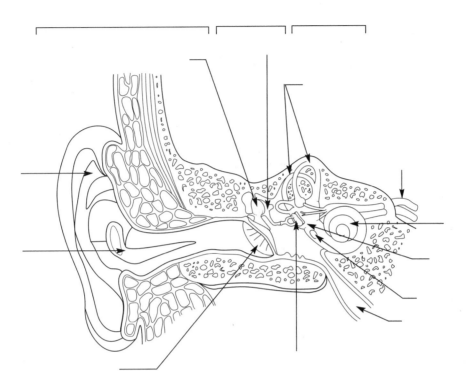

4. Label and color the brain structures in the following figures.

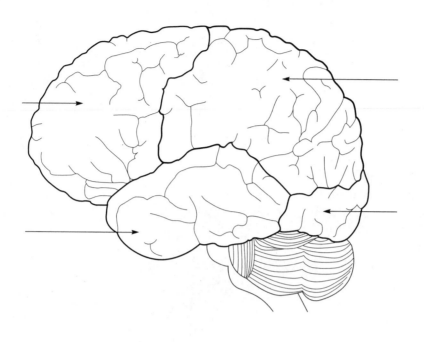

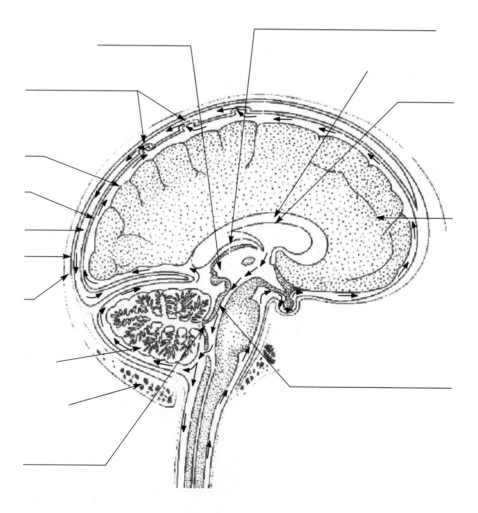

ACTIVITIES

1. Examine a real human skull; then identify all of the structures referred to in the textbook. Take special note of the delicate structures within the nasal cavity. Locate the sinuses.

_____

_____

_____

_____

_____

2. Examine the structures inside a real, preserved eye. Dissect a cow or sheep eye if possible. Identify as many parts as possible. What are the differences in the animal's eye compared to the human eye?

_____

_____

_____

_____

_____

3. Examine the eyes and ears of another student in the class. Use a magnifying glass or otoscope/ophthalmoscope if available.

_____

_____

_____

_____

_____

ONLINE RESEARCH

■ Research current theories on how the brain stores memories. Explain how the mechanism described can be disrupted by head injuries that cause some type of amnesia.

_____

_____

_____

_____

_____

■ Research the current theories on how sleep, or lack of sleep, affects performance. Discuss how these theories can be applied to athletics.

_____

_____

_____

_____

CHAPTER 24

The Spine

(continues)

KEY CONCEPTS

- The nervous system uses electrical impulses, which travel along the length of the cells, to initiate action.
- The peripheral nervous system connects the central nervous system to various body structures. The autonomic nervous system is a specialized portion of the peripheral nervous system that controls the involuntary activities of the vital organs.
- The sympathetic system consists of nerves that extend to all internal vital organs. This system prepares the body to respond to an external stimulus that it perceives as dangerous; this is the fight or flight response.
- Neck injuries can be very serious, so proper management is critical. If a neck injury is suspected, do not move the athlete. It is very important to maintain the athlete's airway. To open the airway, use the jaw-thrust technique. If the athlete is wearing a helmet, do not remove it; a face mask can be cut away to allow access to the airway. Once the airway has been opened and is managed, check for pulse. The spine should be manually immobilized to keep the athlete from moving the head and causing further injury. EMS should be activated.
- A ruptured or herniated disk will usually be characterized by severe pain; stiffness in the lower back; pain in the buttocks; and unilateral radiating leg pain, if the compression of the spinal cord is severe. Associated signs may include muscle weakness, sensory loss, or loss of reflexes in the legs.
- Athletic competition produces tremendous forces and stresses on the spine that can cause injury. Common injuries to the spine include:
  - Cervical spine injuries, which range in severity from neck pain to paralysis. Very serious cervical spine injuries can also result in death. These are emergency situations; special care must be taken when managing and treating an athlete with a cervical spine injury so as not to make the injury worse.
  - Cervical sprains and strains, the most common neck injuries. These types of injuries vary in severity. Injuries of this nature should be checked by a physician.
  - Cervical fracture and subluxation, which are breakage or dislocation of the structures of the spine. These injuries are not common.
  - Thoracic spine injuries, such as contusions, sprains, and strains. These injuries should be treated by a physician.

(continues)

(continued)

- Lumbar spine injuries, usually consisting of contusions, sprains, and strains. These injuries should be treated by a physician.
- Spondylolysis, the breakdown of structures of the spine. This is often attributed to overuse.
- Intervertebral herniated disk, which is the displacement of the material inside the disk so that it presses against the spinal cord. This condition should be treated by a physician.
- Sacroiliac injuries, which are usually sprains resulting from acute or chronic trauma.

OUTLINE

I. The Nervous System
A. The nervous system collects information about external and internal conditions, analyzes that information, then initiates the appropriate response aimed primarily toward survival needs.
    1. The brain and spinal cord make up the central nervous system.
    2. The nervous system's other division is called the peripheral nervous system. The autonomic nervous system is a specialized part of the peripheral system that controls the involuntary, or automatic, activities of the vital internal organs.
II. The Peripheral and Autonomic Nervous Systems
A. The peripheral nervous system consists of all nerves and ganglia located outside the brain and spinal cord (central nervous system).
B. Nerves, including the sensory (afferent) nerves, the motor (efferent) nerves, and mixed nerves, carry impulses to and from the brain.
C. The cranial nerves and spinal nerves make up the entire peripheral nervous system.
    1. The cranial nerves provide communication pathways between the head and neck and the brain.
    2. The spinal nerves provide communication pathways between the rest of the body and the spinal cord, which also provides links to the brain.
    3. The spinal nerves form a network, called a plexus.
D. The autonomic nervous system is a subdivision of the peripheral nervous system (cranial and spinal nerves) that controls the involuntary or automatic activities of the body.
    1. The autonomic nervous system is divided into two systems: the sympathetic nervous system, concerned with preparing the body for action ("fight or flight response"), and the parasympathetic nervous system, which counteracts the sympathetic system to prepare the body for more restful activities.
    2. The two systems operate as a pair.
E. Reflexes are the simplest type of nervous response. They are unconscious and involuntary.
    1. As few as two neurons are necessary for a reflex, though many involve three neurons.

2. Every reflex act is preceded by a change in the environment, called a stimulus.

3. Special structures called receptors pick up these stimuli.

4. If two nerves are involved, all that is necessary is a sensory receptor, which is the distal end of the sensory neuron that carries the sensation to the central nervous system. The sensory neuron communicates to a motor neuron through a neurotransmitting chemical diffusing across a synapse.

5. The motor neuron then sends a signal to an effector, which provides the response (usually a muscle contraction or glandular secretion).

III. The Spine

A. The vertebral column is divided into five sections: the cervical vertebrae, which include the atlas and the axis; the thoracic vertebrae that articulate with the ribs; the lumbar vertebrae that bear most of the body's weight; the sacrum, which forms the posterior pelvic girdle and serves as an articulation point for the hips; and the coccyx, which is formed by four fused bones.

B. The spinal cord begins at the base of the skull and continues to the second lumbar vertebra.

1. It is surrounded by the three meninges and cerebrospinal fluid for protection.

2. The spinal cord consists of gray matter internally, which is surrounded by white matter.

a. For reflex action and communication with the brain, neuron connections are made within the gray matter, while the white matter consists of neuron fibers.

IV. Injuries to the Spine

A. Cervical spine injuries can lead to serious problems or death. The most serious injuries are the result of axial loading or cervical compression, which may cause vertebral fracture or the articular facets to slide away from each other.

1. Symptoms includes unconsciousness, numbness, paralysis, and neck pain with movement.

2. Treatment includes airway management using the jaw-thrust technique. If a helmet is worn, do not remove it because the head movements may increase the severity of the injury. Check for the carotid pulse. If absent, begin chest compressions. Immobilize the neck until EMS arrives.

B. Cervical sprains and strains vary in severity.

1. Symptoms include tenderness and pain at the injury site, though neck motion will not be affected. With moderate sprains and strains, there will be limited movement, but without radiation of pain or paresthesia (abnormal sensation). In more severe injuries, there will be localized pain and muscle spasm, and the athlete may complain of an insecure feeling about the neck.

2. Treatment includes protecting the area, exclusion from further athletic activity, and referral to a physician.

C. Cervical nerve syndrome results from forced lateral flexion, which causes the nerve roots to be either stretched or impinged. This condition is commonly called a pinched nerve, burner, or stinger.

1. Symptoms include a sharp, burning, radiating pain. If the brachial plexus is involved, there may be radiating pain, numbness, and loss of function of the arm and possibly hand.

2. Symptoms usually subside in minutes, though it may leave residual soreness and paresthetic (numbness, tingling) areas.

D. Cervical fractures and subluxations (incomplete or partial dislocations) are not common in athletics, but do occur in sports like football, diving, and gymnastics. Most fatal or paralyzing injuries occur when an athlete's neck is in flexion and the athlete receives a blow to the crown of the head.

1. Symptoms include swelling within the spinal cord, transitory paralysis, neck pain, muscle spasms, numbness, loss of sensation, weakness, paresthesia, and partial or complete limb paralysis.

2. Athletes may experience transient quadriparesis or quadriplegia, also called neuropraxia. Recovery usually occurs within a few minutes, but may last 36 to 48 hours. Referral to a physician for further medical attention is necessary.

3. Possible causes of neuropraxia and transient quadriparesis may be spinal stenosis, congenital abnormality, cervical instability, or intervertebral disk herniation.

4. Because most mechanisms causing cervical spine injury involve forces to the head, injuries to the head and neck must be considered together.

E. Thoracic spine injuries include contusions, sprains, and strains.

1. Symptoms include tenderness, spasms, increased pain with active contraction or stretching, and a stiff back.

2. The athlete should be referred to a physician for further evaluation.

F. Lumbar spine injuries can be aggravated by inadequate or inappropriate conditioning, inflexibility, congenital anomalies, and poor postural habits.

1. Contusions are more common in the paraspinal muscles, but may also occur over the subcutaneous spinous processes.

2. Severe injuries are extremely rare in athletics.

G. Spondylolysis is a defect in the pars interarticularis of the vertebrae; if bilateral, it can allow the vertebra to slip forward on the vertebrae of the sacrum, known as spondylolisthesis.

1. Symptoms include complaint of low back pain associated with increased activity and pain radiating into the buttocks and upper thighs.

2. Refer athlete to a physician for diagnosis.

H. With intervertebral disc herniation, the nucleus pulposus herniates, or protrudes, through the annulus fibrosus and presses against the spinal cord or spinal nerve roots.

1. Symptoms include extreme pain and stiffness in the lower back, pain in the buttocks, and radiating leg pain, if the compression is severe. The leg pain is usually unilateral and follows the route of the sciatic nerve, with possible unilateral muscle weakness, sensory loss, or reflex loss in the affected leg.

2. Refer athlete to a physician for further evaluation.

I. Sacroiliac injuries are usually sprains as a result of acute or chronic trauma.

1. Symptoms include sacroiliac pain and stiffness and soreness of the sacroiliac joint that diminishes during activity, but returns as the athlete cools down.

VOCABULARY REVIEW

Matching

Match the terms on the right with the definitions on the left. Terms may be used once, more than once, or not at all.

_____ 1. The first cervical vertebra; it articulates with the axis and occipital skull bone

_____ 2. The superior seven bones of the spinal column

_____ 3. The five vertebrae associated with the lower part of the back

_____ 4. Any of three membranes that enclose the brain and spinal cord

_____ 5. Twelve pairs of nerves that begin in the brain and transmit messages to various parts of the face and head to stimulate various functions

_____ 6. The organs that respond to a stimulus

_____ 7. A nerve that carries nerve impulses from the periphery to the central nervous system; also known as a sensory nerve

_____ 8. Rings of collagen fibers that surround the intervertebral disk

_____ 9. A nerve that carries messages from the brain and spinal cord to muscles and glands; also known as a motor nerve

_____ 10. The inner part of the spinal cord and outer part of the brain

_____ 11. Dislocation of a disc, resulting in pressure against the spinal cord

_____ 12. A nerve composed of both afferent and efferent nerve fibers

_____ 13. A division of the autonomic nervous system that prepares the body for action; the fight or flight response

_____ 14. The 12 bones of the spine located in the chest area

_____ 15. A nerve that carries messages from the brain and spinal cord to muscles and glands; also known as an efferent nerve

_____ 16. The body system that consists of the brain and spinal cord

_____ 17. The cessation of function of a nerve without degenerative changes occurring

A. afferent nerve

B. annulus fibrosus

C. atlas

D. autonomic nervous system

E. axis

F. central nervous system

G. cervical nerve syndrome

H. cervical vertebrae

I. cranial nerve

J. effectors

K. efferent nerve

L. gray matter

M. intervertebral disc herniation

N. lumbar vertebrae

O. meninges

P. mixed nerve

Q. motor nerve

R. neuropraxia

S. nucleus pulposus

T. paresthesia

U. parasympathetic system

V. peripheral nervous system

W. plexus

X. quadriparesis

Y. quadriplegia

Z. receptor

AA. reflex

BB. sacroiliac joint

_____ 18. A division of the peripheral nervous system that consists of a collection of nerves, ganglia, and plexuses through which visceral organs, heart, blood vessels, glands, and smooth muscles receive their innervation

_____ 19. An injury to the neck resulting from a forced lateral flexion that causes the nerves to be stretched or impinged

_____ 20. The second cervical vertebra

_____ 21. A gelatin-like substance in the center of the vertebral disc

_____ 22. A sensation of tingling, crawling, or burning of the skin

_____ 23. Any change in the environment

_____ 24. The area just under the skin, over each protrusion of the vertebrae

_____ 25. A division of the nervous system, made up of 12 pairs of cranial nerves and 31 pairs of spinal nerves, that provides a communication link between the body tissues and the central nervous system

_____ 26. A network of spinal nerves

_____ 27. The wedge-shaped bone below the lumbar vertebrae at the end of the spinal column

_____ 28. An involuntary reaction to a stimulus

_____ 29. The area between the sacrum and the pelvis

_____ 30. A division of the autonomic nervous system that inhibits, or opposes, the effects of the sympathetic system

_____ 31. The largest nerve in the body, originating in the sacral plexus, which runs through the pelvis and down the leg

_____ 32. A nerve that carries nerve impulses from the periphery to the central nervous system; also known as an afferent nerve

_____ 33. A sensory nerve that receives a stimulus and transmits it to the central nervous system

_____ 34. One of 31 pairs of nerves originating from the spinal cord

_____ 35. The outer part of the spinal cord and inner part of the brain, composed mostly of nerve fibers

_____ 36. An incomplete or partial dislocation of a joint

_____ 37. On one side only

CC. sacrum
DD. sciatic nerve
EE. sensory nerve
FF. spinal cord
GG. spinal nerve
HH. stimulus
II. subcutaneous spinous process
JJ. subluxation
KK. sympathetic system
LL. thoracic vertebrae
MM. unilateral
NN. white matter

ANATOMY IDENTIFICATION

1. Label all of the spinal nerve plexuses and groups of spinal nerves.

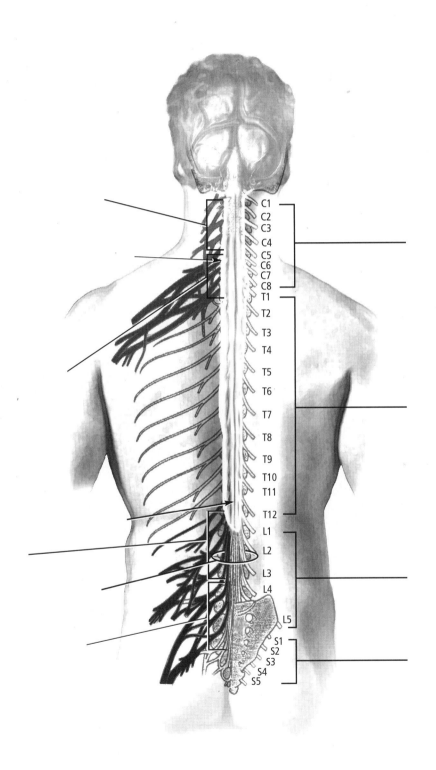

2. Label and color all anatomical areas, including the structures found on the atlas and axis, referred to in the textbook on the following figures.

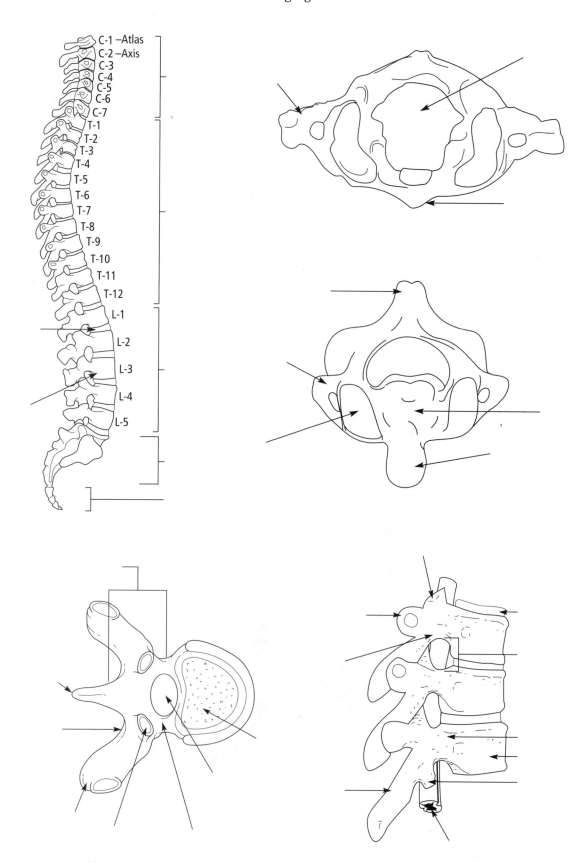

ACTIVITY

1. Examine a model of a spinal column that shows the spinal nerves and spinal cord. Identify all structures referred to in the textbook. Be able to show another person these parts without looking at diagrams or notes.

_____

_____

_____

_____

_____

ONLINE RESEARCH

■ Using the Internet, research what progress is being made to repair severed or partially severed spinal cords. Explain why this is so difficult to do.

_____

_____

_____

_____

_____

CHAPTER 25

Special Considerations in Athletes

KEY CONCEPTS

- Heat exhaustion is a mild form of heat illness characterized by skin that is cool, moist, and pale; generalized weakness; dizziness; and nausea. Fluid replacement and cooling of the body are vitally important at this stage of heat illness. If not treated, heat illness can progress to heatstroke. Heatstroke is a life-threatening form of heat illness characterized by hot, dry, red skin; mental confusion; and unconsciousness. Heatstroke is a medical emergency.

- The body loses heat in five ways: respiration—heat escapes during exhalation; conduction—heat escapes to a cooler surface; evaporation—heat escapes through the skin via perspiration; radiation—heat escapes to the cooler environment; convection—heat escapes to circulated air currents.

- Hyperthermia is a condition in which the body temperature increases above normal. The key to managing hyperthermia is to cool the body. This can be done by moving the athlete to a shaded area, removing any unnecessary clothing, applying cool water to the extremities, fanning the athlete, and giving the athlete cool water to drink.

  Hypothermia is a condition in which the body temperature decreases below normal. The key to managing hypothermia is to warm the body. This can be accomplished by removing the athlete from the cold climate, removing wet or cold clothes, applying warm clothes or a blanket, and providing warm liquids to drink.

- Environmental conditions can greatly affect the health and well being of athletes. During summer sports, pay close attention to the heat index; during winter sports, pay attention to the wind chill. These are both good gauges for determining the risk posed by environmental exposure. At all times, athletes should remain adequately hydrated. This will help protect the athlete from the possible risks of environmental exposure.

- A variety of skin conditions can be caused or made worse by participation in athletics. They are usually caused by bacteria and fungi that thrive in warm, damp areas. Infectious forms of these conditions can spread rapidly from athlete to athlete in contact sports. Skin conditions can be prevented with proper hygiene and ensuring that equipment and shoes fit properly.

- There are two forms of diabetes. Type 1 diabetes results from the body's failure to produce insulin. Individuals with Type 1 diabetes need to maintain blood

(continues)

(continued)

sugar levels within a target range. This is often accomplished through meal planning, exercise, and insulin injections. Type 2 diabetes results from insufficient bodily production of insulin. Type 2 diabetes can be controlled through diet and exercise.

■ Epilepsy is a chronic condition with a variety of causes. However, the ultimate cause of epilepsy is unknown. Seizures resulting from epilepsy can be either partial, affecting only one area of the body, or generalized, affecting the entire body and causing a temporary decrease in the level of consciousness.

■ A systemic reaction is a generalized reaction occurring within just a few minutes of an insect sting or bite. The mildest symptoms are flushed skin and an itchy rash. More serious symptoms include difficulty breathing, nausea, vomiting, palpitations, and fainting. The time of onset indicates the degree of severity of the reaction.

■ Competitive athletes may be at a higher risk than the more casual athlete due to a more rigorous training schedule and the "play-to-win" nature of their sports.

■ The female athlete triad is characterized by disordered eating, amenorrhea, and osteoporosis. Competitive athletes are at a higher risk for the disorder than are more casual athletes. The triad also occurs more often in athletes who participate in sports in which body image is important. Disordered eating can lead to a loss of strength, poor concentration, and additional injuries. Amenorrhea contributes to bone loss and may lead to osteoporosis. Osteoporosis places the athlete at great risk for fractures.

OUTLINE

I. Special Considerations in Athletics

    A. The training staff needs to be aware of any medical condition an athlete has so they can be prepared if an emergency should arise.

II. Environmental Conditions and Athletic Participation

    A. Heat stress occurs when the body cannot maintain homeostasis and the body temperature begins to rise (hyperthermia).

        1. The hypothalamus of the brain is in control of maintaining body temperature (thermoregulation).

        2. Athletes need to be well hydrated, rested, and in good physical condition for temperature regulation to work properly.

        3. The heat index combines temperature and humidity to provide a reference point for various levels of risk associated with exercise under hot and humid conditions.

    B. Dehydration in athletics is usually due to the increased demand for water during exercise, which can be lost by the body at a rate of one to two liters per hour during vigorous exercise.

1. Symptoms are subtle at first, exhibiting light yellow urine, mild headache and fatigue, followed by reduced endurance and oxygen uptake. Then comes a feeling of thirst. Signs of serious dehydration include disorientation, irritability, rapid pulse, and complete exhaustion. There are three levels of dehydration:
   a. Mild involves mucous membranes drying out, normal pulse, yellow urine, mild thirst.
   b. Moderate involves extremely dry mucous membranes, weak and rapid pulse, very dark urine, a very thirsty feeling.
   c. Severe involves completely dry mucous membranes, disorientation, drowsiness, no urine output, inability to form tears, and the beginning stages of shock (rapid weak pulse, rapid breathing, and pale skin).
2. The best treatment is prevention. It is recommended that athletes drink 17 to 20 oz. two to three hours before activity begins, 7 to 10 oz. after warm-up, 28 to 40 oz. every hour of play, and 20 to 24 oz. afterward for every pound of body weight lost through sweat.
3. The use of sports drinks in place of water has been debated for some time. Sports drinks do contain carbohydrates and electrolytes that the body may need, especially for endurance athletes.

C. Sunburns are caused by overexposure to ultraviolet (UV) light from the sun, which can also lead to premature skin aging and skin cancer.
   1. Medical attention should be sought if the burn is severe enough to cause blistering.
   2. Treatment includes application of a cold washcloth and use of an over-the-counter pain medication. Petroleum products should be avoided.
   3. Prevention involves use of sunscreen on exposed skin with a sun protection factor (SPF) of 15 or greater.

D. Heat cramps are common and should not be overlooked because they can be the first stage of heat illness.
   1. Heat cramps occur mostly in the calf muscles, but may affect the quadriceps, hamstrings, and abdominal muscles. They are caused by rapid water and electrolyte loss through perspiration.
   2. Treatment includes slow, passive stretching with application of ice, and immediate fluid and electrolyte replacement.

E. Heat syncope (fainting) occurs when the body tries to cool itself through the dilation of blood vessels.
   1. Symptoms include lightheadedness, dizziness, headache, nausea, and vomiting.
   2. Treatment includes drinking fluids and stopping activity.

F. Heat exhaustion is a condition of near-total body collapse, where the athlete experiences difficulty dissipating the heat.
   1. Symptoms include skin that is cool, moist, and pale, generalized weakness, dizziness and nausea, and rapid breathing and pulse. It may progress to heatstroke if not treated.
   2. Treatment includes moving the athlete to the shade, immediate fluid replacement, and cooling the body, using ice towels if necessary.

G. Heatstroke is the most severe heat-related condition, where the body's heat-regulation mechanism breaks down.

1. Symptoms include hot, dry, red skin and a strong, rapid pulse, with possible mental confusion and unconsciousness.

2. Treatment is to move the athlete to the shade and cool immediately by removing unnecessary clothing and icing with towels with ice packs in the axilla and groin areas. Misting and fanning the skin also helps lower body temperature.

3. Heatstroke is a medical emergency and requires immediate transport to an emergency room by EMS.

H. Cold stress

   1. The body loses heat in five ways.

      a. Respiration rids the body of heat with every expiration.

      b. Evaporation of perspiration and other moisture from the skin causes the body to lose heat.

      c. Conduction occurs when the body is in direct contact with a cooler object. Heat from the body flows to the cooler object; for example, sitting on cool ground or standing or swimming in cool water.

      d. Radiation is the transfer of heat by infrared rays. Just as the body gains heat from the infrared rays of the sun, it can lose heat by infrared rays to a cooler environment.

      e. Convection occurs when heat near the body's surface is removed by moving air, such as wind.

   2. The four factors that contribute to cold stress are cold temperatures, high or cold winds, dampness, and cold water. The body must work harder to maintain its temperature.

   3. Wind chill is the term used to describe the rate of heat loss on the human body resulting from the combined effects of low temperature and wind.

      a. Wind-chill temperature is a measure of relative discomfort due to combined cold and wind, originally developed in 1941 and revised in 2001 to make use of advances in science and technology.

      b. The effects of wind chill depend strongly on the amount of clothing and other protection worn, age, health, and body characteristics. Wind-chill temperatures near or below 0°F indicate a risk of frostbite to exposed flesh.

I. Hypothermia occurs when body heat is lost (from being in a cold environment) faster than it can be replaced.

   1. Symptoms begin when body temperature reaches 95°F. The victim begins shivering and stomping feet to generate heat. As body temperature drops to around 85°F, symptoms include slurred speech, lack of coordination, memory loss, and unconsciousness. Death may occur around 78°F.

   2. People who have experienced trauma often go into shock and begin to shiver, a warning sign of hypothermia. Physical or mental trauma limits the body's capability to regulate its own temperature.

   3. As core body temperature decreases, severe hypothermia sets in.

J. Frostbite occurs when skin tissue and blood vessels are damaged from exposure to temperatures below 32°F. It commonly affects toes, fingers, earlobes, chin, cheeks, and nose.

1. Frostbite occurs in three stages.
   a. Frostnip is a pins-and-needles sensation, and the skin turns very white and soft.
   b. Superficial frostbite may show blistering. The skin is numb, waxy, and frozen, and ice crystals form in the skin cells.
   c. Deep frostbite involves the freezing of blood vessels, muscles, tendons, nerves, and bone. This stage can lead to permanent damage, blood clots, and gangrene. No feeling is experienced in the affected area and there is usually no blistering. Serious infection and loss of limbs is frequent. Medical attention is needed as soon as possible.

2. Emergency care should be provided. If it is not possible to immediately transport to a hospital, the following steps will help:
   a. Bring the individual indoors as soon as possible.
   b. Apply warm towels or immerse the area in circulating lukewarm water for 20 minutes. Leave any blisters intact.
   c. Do not use hot water or hold the affected area near fire.
   d. Offer warm fluids to the athlete, but never alcohol, which causes the blood to cool quickly.
   e. Keep the affected area raised.

III. Skin Conditions in Athletes

A. Acne mechanica is the result of heat, pressure, occlusion, and friction, which usually occur on the shoulders, back, and head, especially when using tight synthetic clothing, such as helmets and shoulder pads. Wearing clean cotton clothing and over-the-counter acne medication is helpful.

B. Plantar warts are small, hard growths on the bottom of the feet which are caused by a virus and are contagious. Treatment, if they don't go away by themselves, includes cutting, burning, freezing (with liquid nitrogen), or treating with chemicals. Not walking barefoot in locker rooms will help prevent the spread of the disease.

C. Herpes gladiatorum is an infection in wrestlers, transmitted through skin-to-skin contact. Treatment is through both topical and oral antifungal medications and exclusion from participation for 10 to 15 days.

D. Fungal infections occur in warm and moist areas of the body, and are commonly referred to as tinea pedis or tinea cruris.
   1. Symptoms include inflammation, burning, itching, scaling, and blistering.
   2. Treatment involves reducing moisture and avoiding transmission.
      a. At home, take off shoes and expose feet to the air.
      b. Change socks and underwear daily.
      c. Dry feet carefully after using a locker room or public shower.
      d. Avoid walking barefoot in public areas.
      e. Do not wear thick clothing for long periods of time in warm weather.
      f. Throw away worn-out exercise shoes, and never borrow other people's shoes.
      g. Do not share towels or headgear.

E. Blisters are caused by friction, along with heat and moisture. A tear occurs, forming a space between layers of the skin with the surface layers intact. Fluid seeps into this space, causing the skin to bubble.

    1. Treatment for athletes involves relieving the pain, keeping the blister from enlarging, and avoiding infection. Care should be taken not to break the skin or pop the blister.

    2. Prevention of blisters involves keeping skin lubricated to reduce friction and reduce moisture. Properly fitting shoes and socks that wick away moisture are critical. Sometimes putting on two pairs of socks and talcum powder before practice helps reduce the chance of getting blisters.

F. Abrasions are common and are normally caused by poorly fitting equipment or rubbing of skin against another athlete or surface. Treat with soap and water, antibiotic cream, and bandaging, which should be replaced daily.

G. Jogger's nipples are caused by friction with clothing, especially during long runs. To prevent this condition, dermatologists recommend applying petroleum jelly, patches, or a bandage over the nipples.

IV. Diabetes

A. Diabetes is a disorder in which the body does not produce or properly use insulin, a hormone that causes body cells to absorb sugar from the blood for use within the cell.

B. Type 1 diabetes results from the body's failure to produce any insulin and usually first appears in childhood to young adulthood. Insulin is normally produced by beta cells within the pancreas. Management of this condition is possible if blood sugar levels are monitored frequently and insulin is injected when necessary.

C. Type 2 diabetes can usually be controlled by diet and exercise because the body still produces insulin, but it is either in insufficient amounts or poorly functioning.

D. Diabetic emergencies are of two types:

    1. Insulin reaction is when there is too much insulin in the body, rapidly reducing the level of sugar in the blood and causing brain cells to suffer.

        a. Insulin reaction can be caused by taking too much medication, failing to eat, heavy exercise, or emotional factors.

        b. Symptoms include fast breathing and pulse, dizziness, weakness, change in the level of consciousness, vision difficulties, sweating, headache, numb hands or feet, and hunger.

        c. Treatment involves giving the athlete sugar if he or she is conscious.

    2. Diabetic coma occurs when there is too much sugar and too little insulin in the blood.

        a. It is caused by eating too much sugar, not taking prescribed medications, stress, or infection.

        b. Symptoms include drowsiness, confusion, deep and fast breathing, thirst, dehydration, fever, a change in the level of consciousness, and a peculiar, sweet- or fruity-smelling breath.

        c. Monitor carefully and seek professional help.

V. Seizure Disorders

A. Seizures are disruptions of normal brain activity.

B. Epilepsy is a condition in which seizures recur regularly.

1. Other causes of seizures include infections, high fever, brain tumors, drugs, strokes, bleeding in the brain, trauma to the brain, and low blood glucose, sodium, or calcium.

2. Epilepsy does not often have a clear cause.

C. A simple partial seizure is when jerking begins in one area of the body, arm, leg, or face. Victims may hear things that are not there, or feel unexplained fear, sadness, anger, or joy. No first aid is necessary, unless the seizure becomes convulsive.

D. A generalized tonic-clonic seizure, or grand mal seizure, is characterized by a sudden cry, falling, and rigidity, followed by muscle jerks, shallow breathing or temporarily suspended breathing, bluish skin, and possible loss of bladder or bowel control.

1. After a couple minutes, normal breathing resumes, though there may still be confusion and/or fatigue.

2. Look for medical identification and protect the victim from nearby hazards. Loosen ties or shirt collars and protect the head from injury. Turn the victim on the side to keep the airway clear, unless an injury exists. If there are multiple seizures, or if one seizure lasts longer than five minutes, call an ambulance.

VI. Insect Bites and Stings

A. The severity and duration of the reaction can vary from person to person. If multiple stings are received or if allergic reactions occur, the situation can be life-threatening.

1. A local reaction is characterized by pain, swelling, redness, itching, and a wheal surrounding the wound.

2. A systemic reaction, if it occurs, happens within a few minutes of a sting and may include skin flushing, an itchy rash, and more seriously, chest wheezing, nausea, vomiting, abdominal pains, palpitations, faintness, falling blood pressure, and death.

3. Epinephrine by injection is the only effective, immediate treatment.

4. An EpiPen is an automatically injecting syringe, designed to inject a premeasured, single dose of epinephrine. It is administered in the front part of the leg through the clothing. Effects will last 15 to 20 minutes. EMS must be activated.

B. Treatment involves:

1. Notifying a companion in case assistance becomes necessary.

2. Immediately removing the sting apparatus by scraping it out of the skin.

3. Applying ice to reduce pain and swelling.

4. Seeking medical assistance if a serious reaction is suspected.

VII. The Female Athlete Triad

A. The female athlete triad involves a combination of three conditions.

1. Disordered eating refers to conditions, such as anorexia and bulimia, that ultimately result in malnutrition.

a. No matter what the sport, if muscles lack sufficient and proper fuel, performance is impaired.

b. Lack of fuel can also lead to inability to concentrate. The athlete with strength losses and poor concentration can be more easily injured.

2. Amenorrhea is the loss of menstrual periods. A certain percentage of body fat in females is necessary for proper functioning of the menstrual cycle. If the body fat percentage gets too low, hormonal balance and the menstrual cycle are affected.

3. Osteoporosis is the loss of bone, most common among women after menopause, whose menstrual cycle also stops functioning. Amenorrhea can lead to osteoporosis in female athletes just like it can in postmenopausal women. Stress fractures become more common and repair is slow.

B. Warning signs of the female athlete triad include:

1. Frequent or unexplained injuries, stress fractures.

2. Excessive or compulsive exercise.

3. Change in performance (loss of endurance, speed, and/or strength).

4. Impaired concentration.

5. Absent or irregular menstrual periods.

6. Restrictive eating masked as a "performance-enhancing" meal plan.

7. Use of weight loss products or supplements.

C. Prevention includes:

1. Choosing an activity that complements an individual's natural body strengths.

2. Realizing health is more important than competitive success.

3. Avoiding frequent weigh-ins, weight comments, and punitive consequences for weight gain.

4. Appreciating a healthy, active body. Optimal weight for health and performance is different for everyone.

5. Realizing that the thinnest athletes are not necessarily the fastest or the strongest.

6. Thinking of fuel as the ultimate performance enhancer.

7. Not starving the bones. Part of the fuel mix should include several servings of good calcium sources.

8. Being a role model with words and actions. Take a positive attitude about fueling and enjoying foods.

VOCABULARY REVIEW

Matching

Match the terms on the right with the definitions on the left. Terms may be used once, more than once, or not at all.

_____ 1. A type of herpes infection, commonly seen in wrestlers

_____ 2. The body's response to too much circulating insulin; the level of sugar in the blood decreases, causing brain cells to suffer

_____ 3. A form of acne seen in athletes as a result of heat, pressure, occlusion, and friction

_____ 4. A life-threatening form of heat illness that involves a rise in body temperature and altered mental status

_____ 5. The inability of the body to maintain homeostasis because of high temperatures

_____ 6. A condition in which there is too much sugar and too little insulin in the blood, resulting in body cells not receiving enough nourishment

_____ 7. A disorder that affects female athletes; characterized by disordered eating, amenorrhea, and osteoporosis

_____ 8. Painful, involuntary muscle spasms caused by exposure to heat and dehydration

_____ 9. The cells of the pancreas responsible for making insulin

_____ 10. The temperature of the human body necessary to maintain homeostasis; 98.6°F.

_____ 11. The mildest form of generalized heat-related illness, characterized by multiple symptoms and often by dehydration

_____ 12. A fungal infection that thrives in warmth and dampness; often referred to as athlete's foot, jock itch, or ringworm

_____ 13. Fainting that occurs when the body attempts to cool itself by dilating the blood vessels

_____ 14. A condition caused by chafing between the runner's nipples and the shirt

_____ 15. Pain, swelling, redness, itching, and formation of a wheal at the site of an insect bite

A. acne mechanica

B. beta cells

C. core body temperature

D. diabetic coma

E. female athlete triad

F. generalized tonic-clonic seizure

G. heat cramps

H. heat exhaustion

I. heat index

J. heat stress

K. heatstroke

L. heat syncope

M. herpes gladiatorum

N. insulin reaction

O. jogger's nipples

P. local reaction

Q. plantar warts

R. simple partial seizure

S. systemic reaction

T. tinea cruris

U. tinea pedis

V. wind chill

_____ 16. Small, hard growths that occur on the bottom of the foot

_____ 17. A type of seizure in which a jerking motion begins in one part of the body, but the victim remains awake and aware

_____ 18. A type of seizure characterized by a sudden cry and falling, rigidity, jerking of muscles, shallow breathing, and loss of bladder and bowel control, usually lasting for a couple of minutes

_____ 19. The rate of heat loss on the human body, resulting from the combined effects of cold temperatures and wind

_____ 20. A reference point indicating the risk associated with outdoor exercise, based upon the calculation of air temperature combined with relative humidity

_____ 21. A generalized reaction to a bug bite, characterized by flushing of the skin and an itchy rash; more serious symptoms such as wheezing, nausea, vomiting, palpitations, and faintness can also occur

_____ 22. A fungal infection found in the groin area

Crossword Puzzle

Identify the terms described in the puzzle clues, then write the letters in the boxes. (Many terms are more than one word.)

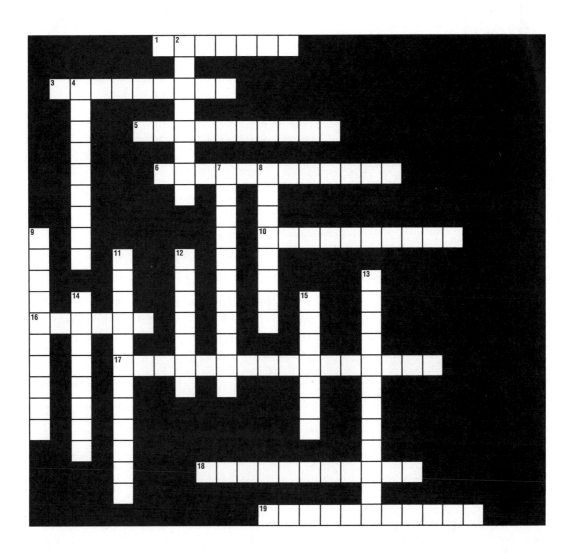

Across

1. disruption in normal brain activity
   _____

3. damage to skin and blood vessels from temperatures below 32°F _____

5. lack of menstrual flow _____

6. bone loss _____

10. heat that is transferred to a cooler object _____

16. an auto-injecting device for epinephrine _____

17. the process of maintaining body temperature _____

18. body temperature is lower than normal _____

19. a state of balance in the body _____

Down

2. seizures that occur regularly throughout life _____

4. heat loss through infrared rays _____

7. heat loss from perspiration _____

8. the organ that produces insulin _____

9. heat loss from the wind blowing past the body _____

11. body temperature is above normal _____

12. overexposure to the sun's UV light _____

13. the temperature-regulating structure in the brain _____

14. when the body does not produce enough insulin _____

15. a hormone that causes cells to absorb glucose from the blood _____

ACTIVITY

1. Construct a poster-sized diagram of a cross section of the skin. Label the names of each part and briefly describe their functions.

_____

_____

_____

_____

_____

ONLINE RESEARCH

■ Many athletes spend a great deal of time in the sun during practice and competitions. This makes them susceptible to skin cancer if protective measures are not taken. Research malignant melanoma on the Internet to find current statistics on its occurrence, treatment, and success of treatment.

_____

_____

_____

_____

_____

■ Research recent heat-related deaths that have occurred among athletes. Discuss conditions that contributed to the difficulty the body had regulating its own body temperature. Identify corrections that were made to prevent this from happening in the future.

_____

_____

_____

_____

_____